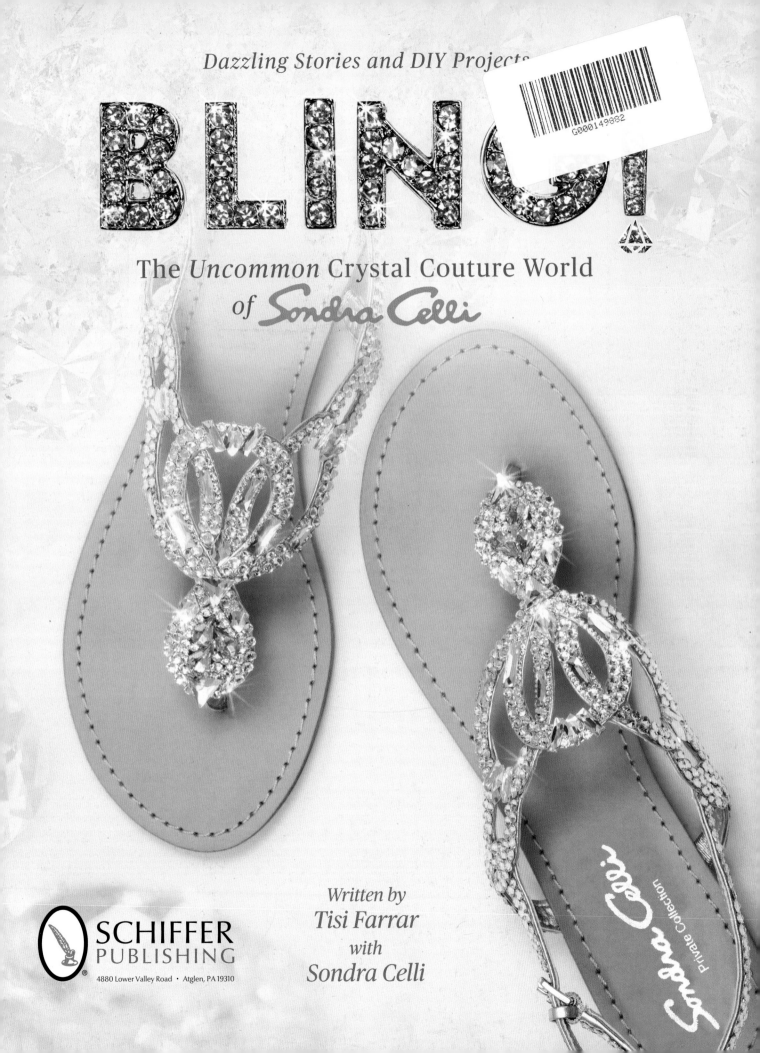

Dazzling Stories and DIY Projects

BLING!

The *Uncommon* Crystal Couture World
of *Sondra Celli*

Written by
Tisi Farrar
with
Sondra Celli

SCHIFFER
PUBLISHING
4880 Lower Valley Road · Atglen, PA 19310

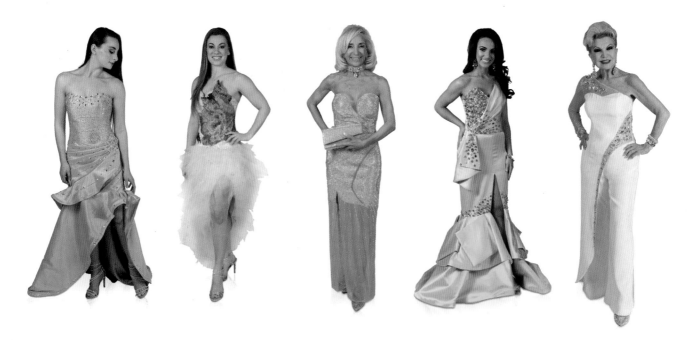

Designed by Danielle D. Farmer
Cover design by Danielle D. Farmer
Type set in illusias/Publico/Avenir LT Std
Back cover flap: Tisi Farrar photo courtesy of Rachael Lynsey Rubin
Diamonds on white background. 3D render top front view © WhiteBarbie. Courtesy of Shutterstock
Silver glitter texture abstract background for design © 4 Girls 1 Boy, Elegant teal turquoise and aqua mint green glitter sparkle confetti background or party invitation for Christmas or birthday with white space © Stephanie Zieber. Courtesy of Big Stock Images

ISBN: 978-0-7643-5733-6
Printed in China

Published by Schiffer Publishing, Ltd.
4880 Lower Valley Road
Atglen, PA 19310
Phone: (610) 593-1777; Fax: (610) 593-2002
E-mail: Info@schifferbooks.com
Web: www.schifferbooks.com

For our complete selection of fine books on this and related subjects, please visit our website at www.schifferbooks.com. You may also write for a free catalog.

Schiffer Publishing's titles are available at special discounts for bulk purchases for sales promotions or premiums. Special editions, including personalized covers, corporate imprints, and excerpts, can be created in large quantities for special needs. For more information, contact the publisher.

We are always looking for people to write books on new and related subjects. If you have an idea for a book, please contact us at proposals@schifferbooks.com.

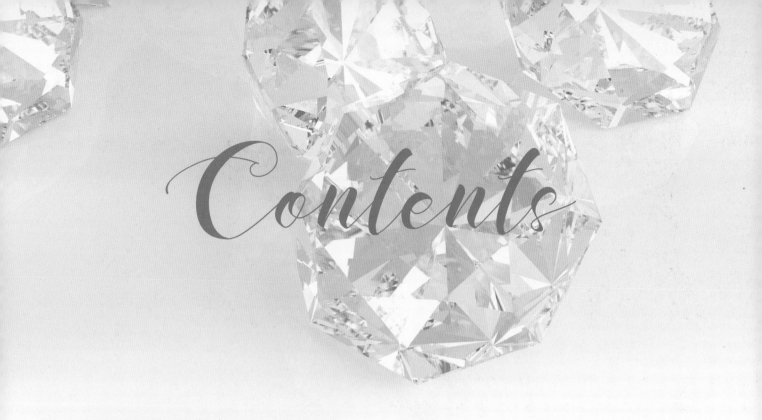

Contents

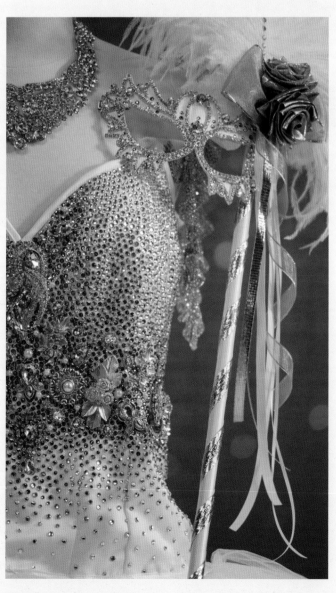

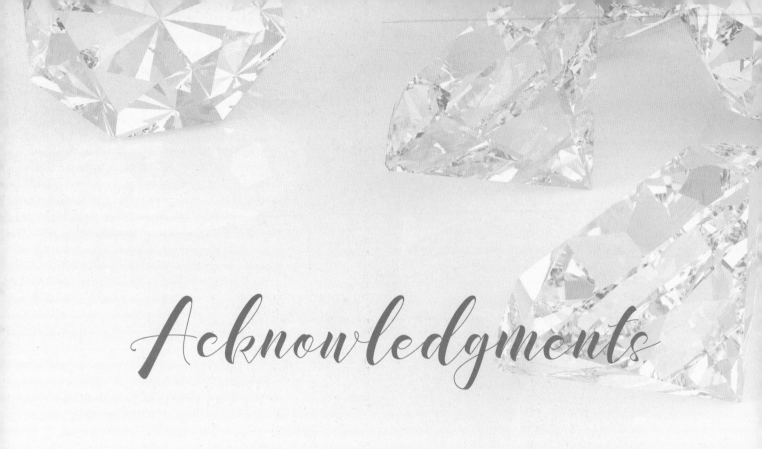

Acknowledgments

Inspiration comes to lots of people, but without support it fades away. Thanks, Mom and Dad, for your love and unwavering commitment to help me to live out my dream.

You bring light and vision into my sparkling world. You are my most brilliant jewel. Thanks, Milan!

Thank you, Tisi Farrar, for all you do behind the scenes and for all the hours you invested in collaborating with me on this book.

Thanks, Mark Johnson, for your photographic skills and boundless energy over the course of countless shoots. You did a brilliant job capturing the bling.

Thanks, Diane Parry and Jay Dwyer, for always being around to lend a helping hand on a moment's notice.

Thank you to my fans. I do read all your letters and postings and truly appreciate your support!

Finally, to the Bling-ettes and my entire staff, a great big and blingy "thank you!" for your dedication, inspiration, creativity, late-night hours, and unmatched artistry. I couldn't do it without you.

–Sondra Celli

Thank you, Sondra Celli, for sharing your art of bling and for your friendship. Working with you is a daily adventure. Your talent is mind-blowing, your creativity is limitless, and your passion for design is unmatched. You put your heart and soul into every piece you make so that each and every client's dream design is beyond realized.

I now know what grows on a book farm. A family. Thank you to our brilliant team of expert editors and skillful designers at Schiffer Publishing who made this book possible. It was an absolute pleasure working with every one of you.

Thank you, Marlowe Farrar, for your patience, tech expertise, and support. You are the L.O.M.L.!

–Tisi Farrar

Preface

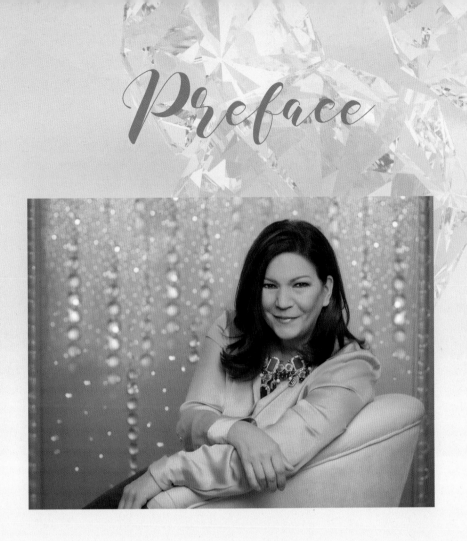

I t has been almost forty years since I started working as a fashion designer, and to this day I am still passionate about what I do.

Designing is creative, exciting, surprising, demanding, and truly rewarding. My clients come from all walks of life and in every age, shape, and size. People come to me when they want to order special outfits to wear to special occasions. I design for brides, mothers of the brides, toddlers, pageant contestants, ballroom dancers, and anyone else searching for that one-of-kind design. Every piece I make is different except for one element that they all have in common, and that is "bling."

Throughout the book I use that word to refer to shimmering crystals: faceted stones that sparkle. To be more specific, the great majority of my work is adorned with genuine Swarovski® bling, which is the best there is. The crystals (also called stones) are unmatched when it comes to sparkle, and they infuse designs with a dynamic radiance. My custom crystal couture can be lightly trimmed or fully packed, but no matter what the quantity of stones requested, the results are always dramatic.

These days the demand for bling is greater than ever. You can find the dazzling stones adorning almost every type of clothing and plenty of other products as well. People can't seem to get enough. I receive countless questions from fans wanting me to teach them how to do what I do, so that they can embellish their own wardrobe.

That's how this book came about. After many years of answering questions, I decided to lay it all out for you fans of bling. In this book I teach you several of the bling techniques that are used in my shop, and walk you through some basic projects you can do at home to polish your skills. As we go, I'll also share some of my life experiences as a designer and behind-the-scenes stories–both good and bad–of the business of bling and of shooting a reality TV show. You can also order my Sondra Celli Bling Kit at a discount with the purchase of this book. The kit comes with a bling tool, Beacon Adhesive's Power-Tac®, stones, instructions, and more of what you need to add bling to your wardrobe (see page 110 for details).

I believe anyone can learn to embellish, with a little patience and a lot of practice. So, come with me now and let's "bling it on" together!

Sondra Celli

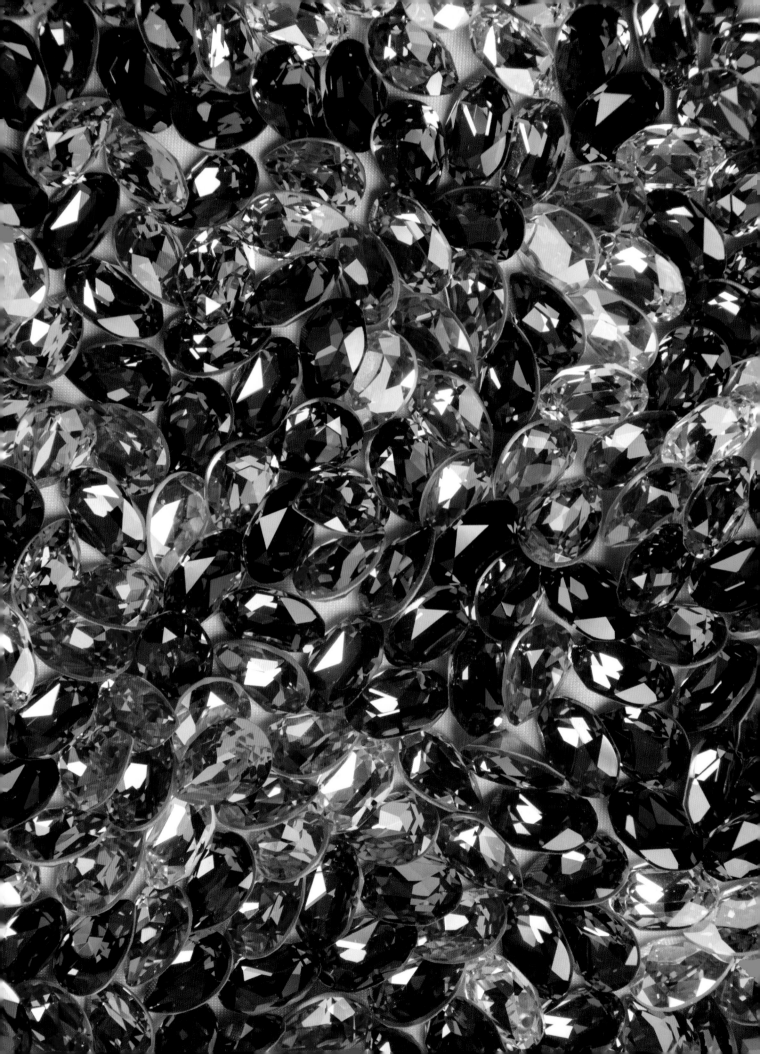

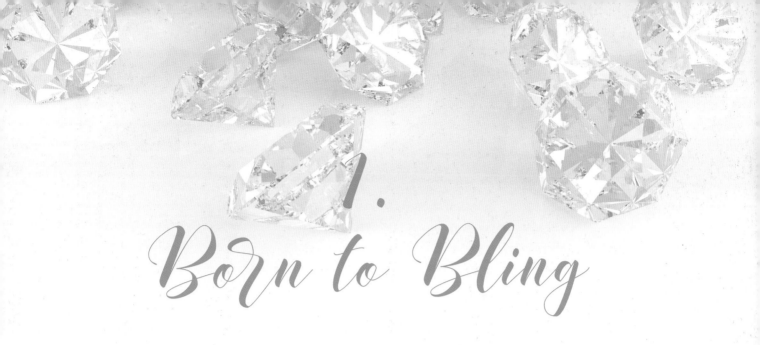

1.
Born to Bling

It was late in the evening before a big fashion show benefit that my mother, Yolanda, was producing. Mom owned a high-end bridal boutique, beauty salon, and health spa all under one roof, called Yolanda's. It was renowned throughout New England for its expansive collection of sparkling designer gowns, bridal dresses, glittery ensembles, and alluring accessories. Several times throughout the year Mom would put on spectacular fashion shows to benefit local charities. Her shows were over-the-top productions featuring glamorous couture from the boutique, outrageous theatrical props, and celebrity models. They always sold out, and tomorrow's event was no exception.

Things were frantic at the shop as the staff ran around doing last-minute packing for our early-morning setup at the venue. I was in the backroom trying to finish up the finale piece. Most couture fashion shows usually end with a fantasy bridal gown, and I was very excited about mine. However, things weren't going well. The skirt kept caving in under the weight of 200 handmade flowers embellished with pearls and beading I had trailing down the dress. The petticoat underneath was useless, providing little support. Removing the flowers was not an option. A lot of time, work, and expense had gone into making them, and they were what made the dress stand out. I was frustrated and stressed out.

My dad, Dan, who was helping pack up props, popped his head into the backroom and asked how I was doing. I told him about my design dilemma and asked if he could think of some way to support the skirt. Dad was a mechanical contractor who ran a successful business.

He was also very creative and could build marvelous things with whatever materials he had on hand. He made displays for Mom's boutique, designed fanciful props for her elaborate fashion shows, and created forts, dollhouses, and tree houses for my younger sister, Linda, and me when we were growing up. When I eventually established my own company, I would often call Dad up to ask his advice on technical design issues.

Dad looked the buckling dress over for several minutes, said he'd be right back, and left. What could he have in mind? Whatever it was, I hoped it would work because I was exhausted and desperately needed sleep. The next thing I knew, Dad walked in carrying a coil of white tubing. He had gone to his truck to retrieve some flexible PVC he had purchased at the hardware store. Dad thought that using it to create a more structured crinoline would help provide the additional support needed to prevent the skirt from caving. It worked perfectly!

The standing-room-only fashion show was a smashing success, as was my finale piece. Who knew I'd be shopping at hardware stores for design elements? Another time I made a ball gown that had to light up. Dad helped again by creating special hoops that could be wired with tiny lights. The lights shone through the opaque overskirt and gave the design a fairy-tale princess glow. I hid the battery packs for the lights in a secret pocket sewn into the skirt. Although Dad is retired now, I can still count on him to be there anytime I need his expert help.

I am often asked how I became a crystal couture designer creating custom ensembles and accessories embellished with bling. It was certainly a family affair.

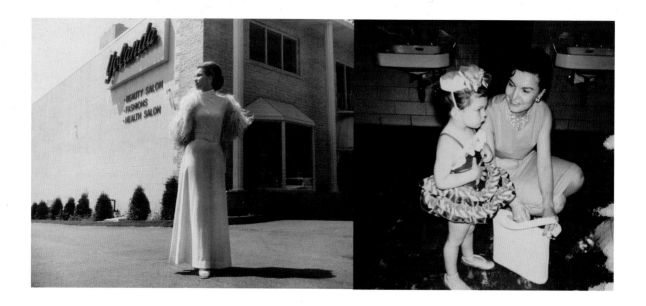

Mom is often referred to as the "Goddess of Glitz," not just for the ornate inventory at Yolanda's, but for her personal style. She always looks like she has just walked off a couture runway–very chic and always glitzy. She adores bling and has never met a sequin, bead, crystal, or pearl she doesn't like. While I was growing up, Mom always used to say she loved bling so much she would sprinkle it on her cereal every morning. My younger sister, Linda, and I often joked that we could always find Mom by following the trail of rhinestones and sequins she left behind.

The apple doesn't fall far from the tree. Although I don't wear a lot of bling, I love using shimmering embellishments for my clothing lines. Today, genuine Swarovski® crystals are the number one design element used in my workroom. They are my favorite kind of bling because they look good on everyone and anything, they add life and movement to designs, they never go out of style, and they grab attention.

Because Mom and Dad both ran their own companies, Linda and I were dropped off at our grandparents' house every day after school. "Nana" would babysit for us until Mom finished her day and came by to pick us up. One of my earliest and fondest childhood memories was sitting with Nana, a naturally gifted handcrafter, who taught me to sew, knit, needlepoint, and crochet. Although Linda wasn't as enthusiastic about our daily lessons, I couldn't get enough and went at them with a passion.

Nana was my mother's mother. Her family immigrated to the United States from Italy when she was just a child. The family was so poor that Nana had to quit school to get a job and help with the family's finances. She received only

Left Publicity photo of Mom standing outside her noted bridal salon, Yolanda's. My contractor father designed and built it for her. 1973. *Courtesy of Yolanda Cellucci*

Right Mom is always glamorously dressed and never leaves the house without makeup on and hair perfectly coifed. Here she is with me at my dance recital in 1961. *Courtesy of Yolanda Cellucci*

Opposite I designed these two gowns for Mom's eightieth birthday celebration. Her dress features gold jewelry pieces and crystal embellishments. The display gown is my "tribute in crystals" to Mom's fashion career: the hemline boasts a couture hat, Mom's celebrated Excalibur limo, and Diamond, her pet Maltese. 2014. *Courtesy of David Fox Photographer*

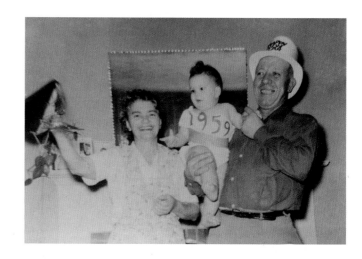

My very first sewing instructor, Nana (Mary DiDuca), me, and Papa (Ralph DiDuca) ring in the New Year, 1959. *Courtesy of Yolanda Cellucci*

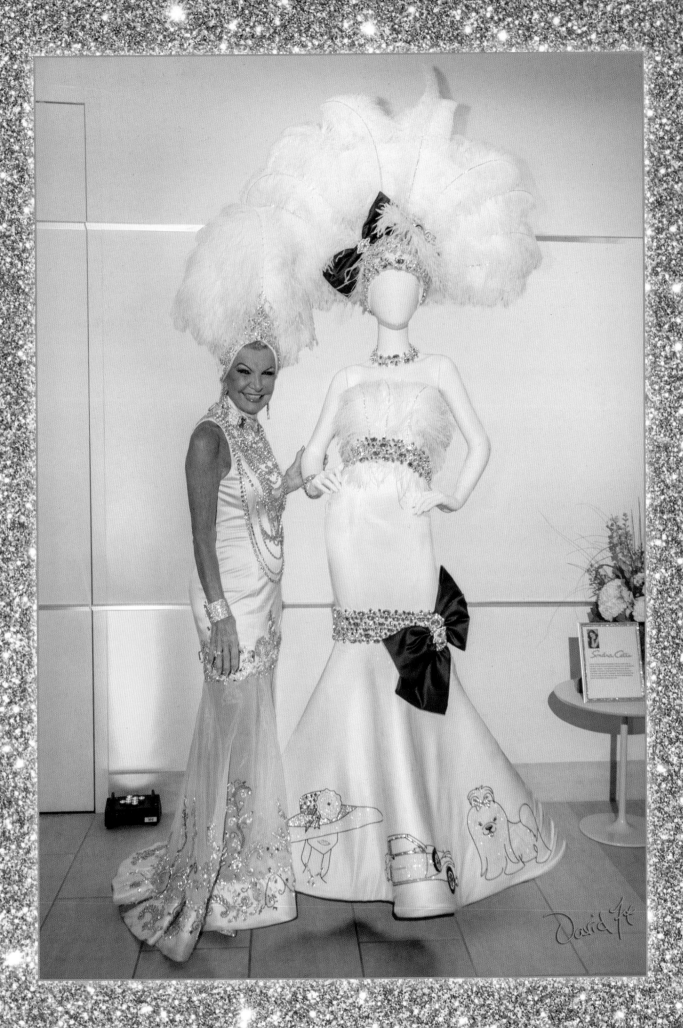

a fifth-grade education and never learned to read. As a result, she couldn't use patterns. Instead, Nana would take apart a blouse or skirt, carefully study its construction, and then re-create patterns from the individual pieces to make clothes. That's exactly how she taught me, and her lessons proved invaluable. Under her loving direction I would spend hours making patterns, cutting, sewing, designing, and embellishing. My wardrobe grew, as did my talent, but the best thing was, Nana allowed me complete creative freedom. It was thrilling to be able to choose my own fabrics and whatever embellishments I wanted to create my own unique designs.

When I turned eight, Nana and Papa presented me with a Singer Golden Touch & Sew sewing machine. I was so excited and got right to work designing a party dress for my big birthday celebration. I created a pink knit jumper and, although every seam was crooked, I was quite impressed with my work. From that day on you could find me sewing up new pieces to add to my ever-expanding wardrobe.

Another one of my early designs was truly original–but for the wrong reason. I made a simple dress by using fabric featuring a pattern packed with tiny sailboats. When I finished my nautical couture, however, all the boats were sailing upside down, resembling submarines. I was not at all deterred by this artistic mishap and kept on designing.

Crystal Clear

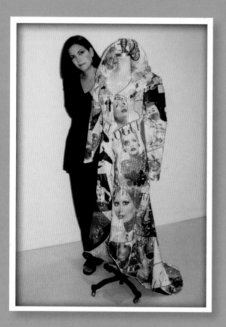

I have worked with lots of quirky items over the years. I have used feather dusters, tea bags (for dyeing white lace ivory), and PVC tubing, as mentioned earlier. One time, while on deadline to finish a gown for my mother, I realized I lacked an extra-long zipper to finish it off. It was two o'clock in the morning, so fabric stores weren't open. What was I to do? I looked around the workroom and found a solution. Grabbing one of my garment bags, I proceeded to rip out the zipper and sew it into the dress. It worked beautifully, don't you agree?

I created this gown by photocopying *Vogue* magazine covers onto fabric, then embellishing them with Swarovski® crystals. The dress was worn by Mom with a matching headpiece when she hosted a benefit fashion show. 1998. *Courtesy of Yolanda Cellucci*

Crystal Clear

As a child I was constantly browsing through fashion magazines. I remember one time finding a picture of a pink sheath dress that I fell head over heels in love with. I decided to make one for myself. The end result was pretty good but far too plain for my taste. It needed a little embellishing. I settled on two of Mom's feather dusters and started pulling them apart. The feather accents were just what the dress needed (and my mother needed two new feather dusters).

When I wasn't sewing, knitting, or crocheting, I used to chop up the Sears catalog and create collages of fashion lines I dreamed about one day manufacturing. Many of those inspired lines were eventually turned into actual pieces for my collection of Barbie dolls. I used fabric remnants, old towels, and any other materials I could scrounge up. I guess I was "recycle cool" before it was cool.

From the very beginning, Mom was one of my biggest fans–and still is. She loves my embellished fashions and even has me add bling to pieces from her personal wardrobe. When I was in sixth grade I told my mom that I didn't want to be transported back and forth to Nana's house anymore. I wanted to stay home after school and spend more time designing for my dolls. It was becoming too much of a chore to pack up all the "gals," plus the assorted fabrics, notions, and embellishments necessary to keep my collection of dolls in custom Celli threads. Knowing how much I loved designing, Mom searched for a new babysitter who could mind us at home but also continue my sewing instruction. Thankfully, she found Patty, who tutored me on how to work with patterns. By combining Nana's informal teaching methods with Patty's more structured techniques, I continued honing my design skills over the next few years.

In seventh grade I had to wear a uniform to school, which I absolutely hated. It was made with fabric that I described as a "sad plaid." To my eye, the colors were dull and needed more pizzazz. I went to work with a bunch of magic markers and colored in different areas of the plaid to give it more life. My mother wasn't happy with my handiwork and neither were school officials when I showed up in my newly altered uniform. Not one to conform, I was transferred out of parochial school and into the public school system within the year.

At my new high school I immediately signed up for a sewing course. My enthusiasm, however, was short-lived when I learned that class assignments were rigidly structured. Apparently, every student was required to make the same design, using only fabrics selected by the instructor. The class was creatively stifling, which brought out my rebellious nature. One assignment called for us to make a jumper, and, as dictated, everyone was issued the same fabric. Breaking from the rigid guidelines, I decided to use a fabric of my own choosing rather than the one issued. As a result, I received a "D" from the instructor with the admonishment that I would never make it in the world of fashion. I guess that "D" stood for determined, since I have been designing now for almost forty years.

Although my creativity was often crushed at school, I found complete creative freedom after school when I began working at my mom's boutique. Every day after school I would head over to Mom's salon, do my homework in the backroom, and then work on alterations. I would shorten or lengthen hems, take in or let out seams, and add beads, fringe, sequins, crystals, and other embellishments.

Because Mom's inventory consisted of high-end designer clothing and accessories, it provided great technical training for me. I studied the impeccable and often-complicated construction of gowns and learned how to work with luxurious fabrics and every kind of trim and beading. I also saw how the various embellishments were applied and how each could enhance a design, transforming it into something sparkle-tacular. When I look back I realize how privileged I was to be able to study

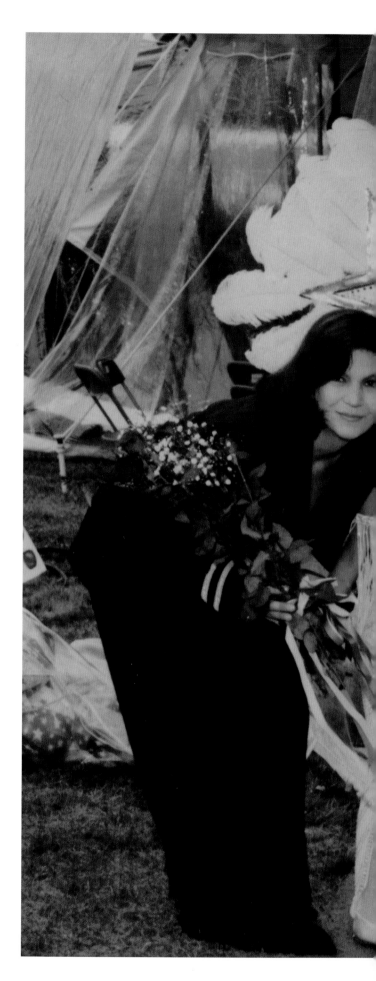

Backstage at one of Mom's elaborate shows. They were always a family affair. Mom was the mistress of ceremonies, I helped design, and Linda and the kids modeled. *Left to right*: me; my daughter, Milan; my nephew, Dimitri; Mom; my nephew, Alec; and Linda. 1996. *Courtesy of Yolanda Cellucci*

design in a real work environment while also learning from my mom how to run and promote a business. The experience was priceless.

Eventually Mom started taking me with her on buying trips to New York City and let me help order inventory for her store. In addition, I began creating original embellished designs for Mom, who would wear them to black-tie events or on stage whenever she hosted her standing-room-only shows. The shows featured sparkling gowns, elaborate headpieces, and Broadway-style props. The entire family was involved. I designed, Dad helped build or source props and load in and out, and Linda modeled. Linda infused every ensemble with life as she strutted confidently down the runway. She was such a pro and very much in demand.

Backstage at fashion shows it's usually chaotic and wardrobe changes have to happen fast. Once when Linda had been hired to work a show for a designer, she walked out wearing his dress backward. When the designer mentioned it during his commentary, Linda never missed a beat. She continued walking the runway while nonchalantly (and expertly) pulling her arms inside the dress, turning it completely around so that the dress was on properly, and, pushing her arms back into the sleeves, did one final turn and walked off. The audience went wild with applause. Linda became a very successful model, gracing numerous magazine covers and appearing in newspaper ads as well as on TV.

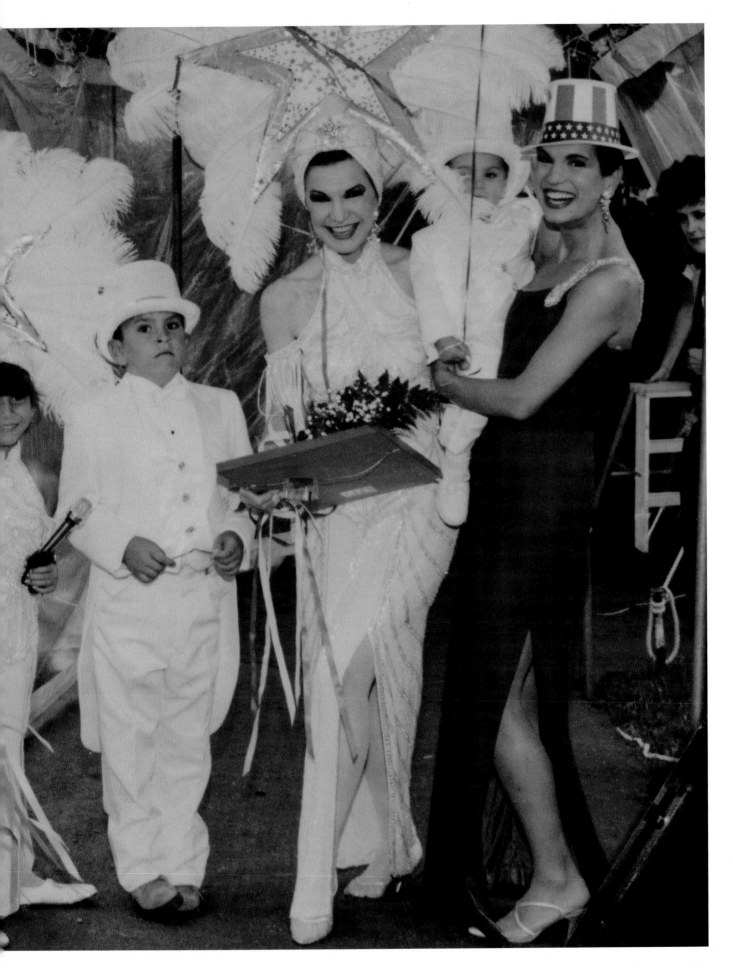

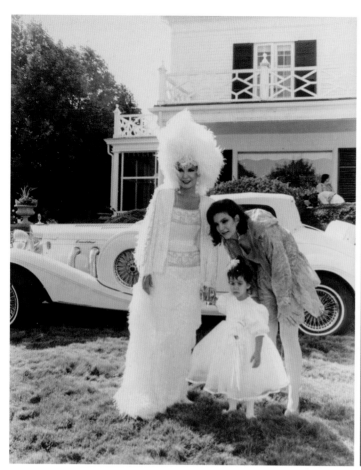

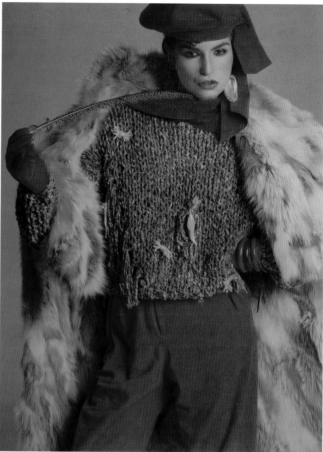

My mom oversaw all aspects of her business: staffing, buying, selling, and promoting. When she was just starting out with her business, she didn't have the money to pay for ads, so she found other ways to promote her business that didn't cost a dime. A great example of that was when she would book a dinner reservation at some popular restaurant on a busy Saturday night and get dressed up in a glamorous gown with lots of bling. She would work it out ahead of time for one of her girlfriends to call up the restaurant and ask to have her paged. When the maître d' came through, asking out loud, "Is there a Ms. Yolanda here?" or "Phone call for Ms. Yolanda," Mom would get up from the table and take her time walking through the entire dining room to the telephone, making sure that all eyes were on her dazzling duds. Staging this event at popular hot spots around Boston caused a lot of buzz and brought glamour-seeking customers to Mom's boutique.

My family and I were all thriving in the family business of fashion and glamour and loved every glitzy moment of it.

Left On location with Mom and Milan standing in front of Mom's Excalibur limo, which was used as a prop. 1992. *Courtesy of Yolanda Cellucci*

Right Linda models one of my early tops in an ad for my women's knitwear collection. 1980. *Courtesy of Sondra Celli*

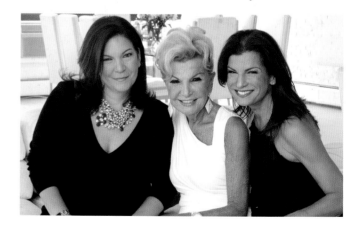

The three fashionistas! *Left to right*: fashion designer (me), fashion entrepreneur (Mom), and fashion cover girl (Linda). 2015. *Courtesy of Tracy Aiguier*

2.
Early Days of Bling

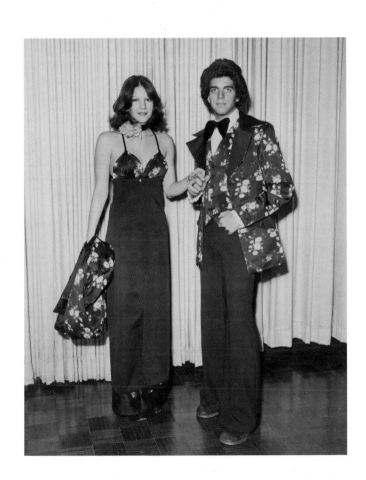

Two memorable events occurred in high school that helped to solidify my dream of becoming a designer. One was meeting an early supporter of my dreams, Mr. Richard O'Neil. He taught a merchandising class that provided the foundation on which to build sales experience. He believed in my talents and encouraged me to enter retail competitions across the country.

The other event was taking advantage of an exchange program to study abroad. During my sophomore year I enrolled in a fantastic summer program that would help steer me directly into my future career path.

This was no ordinary program: called "Food, Fashion, and Furnishings," it was the perfect fit for me. I traveled to different countries while studying the business of retail, manufacturing, and fashion, as well as exploring the food, fashion, and furnishings of each country. During the day I took classes on design concepts, how commerce works, and culture, while afternoons were left free for exploring.

In Italy, I studied the businesses of designer Emilio Puccio; in England, the focus was on Biba and Mary Quant cosmetics. In France, I studied Christian Dior and took classes at the renowned Cordon Bleu cooking school. My studies continued in Sweden with a focus on George Jensen Silver Forge, in Denmark it was Royal Doulton and Birger Christensen Furs, and in Switzerland it was a delicious mix of chocolate and cheese factories.

As a student of fashion, of course I designed my prom date's tuxedo to coordinate with my custom floral satin gown. I guess the tux was a hit, since this photo appeared in the window of a local tuxedo shop the very next day. 1975. *Courtesy of Sondra Celli*

I returned from Europe knowing wholeheartedly that I wanted to be a designer. As a senior in high school, I now needed to focus on my next steps towards achieving a design degree. That's when I discovered New York City's Fashion Institute of Technology (FIT) and enthusiastically applied for admission. I was ecstatic when I received my official acceptance letter and started packing before I had even picked up my high school diploma. I spent the next two years pursuing design knowledge while taking advantage of various internships to gain invaluable experience. I interned at a pattern company, Papaleo Pattern, where I hand cut patterns and learned to grade up sizes by hand, since computer programs for that didn't exist at the time. "Grading up" meant creating a series of patterns increasing in size by fractions of inches, to give you a variety of fits such as XS, S, M, L, and XL. These were then used to make garments to fit men, women, and children of all sizes.

At FIT, my focus of study was menswear, because I wanted to learn tailoring. In 1976, I graduated with my degree and the dream of one day opening a menswear store of my own.

My first paid job after graduation was at Bon Homme Shirt Company, where I worked as an assistant designer creating disco shirts. Some of you may remember those once-popular polyester tops featuring wild patterns that men wore, usually unbuttoned to the navel and accented with heavy gold neck chains. I am sure I am not the only one who was thankful when those shirts went out of style.

From Bon Homme I moved on to a job at Piedmont Industries, a company producing lines for Pierre Cardin, Oleg Cassini, and the Sears Winnie-the-Pooh collection, among others. While there I was responsible for designing men's big and tall shirts and boys' sportswear. Next, I accepted a freelance job designing a high-end knit line of women's sweaters for Emilio Rossi based in Prato, Italy, as well as a mid-priced line to be produced in Hong Kong.

Below Early design layouts of my spring/summer lines for Piedmont Industries' boyswear division. 1980. *Courtesy of Sondra Celli*

Opposite top My mentor, Richard O'Neil. 1976. *Courtesy of Sondra Celli*

Opposite bottom My dad looking dapper in a gray velvet tuxedo jacket with gray flannel vest and pants I designed for him. 1978. *Courtesy of Yolanda Cellucci*

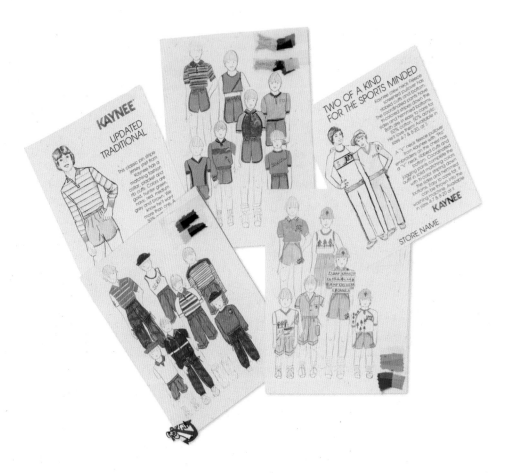

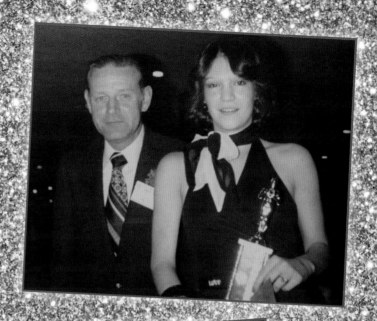
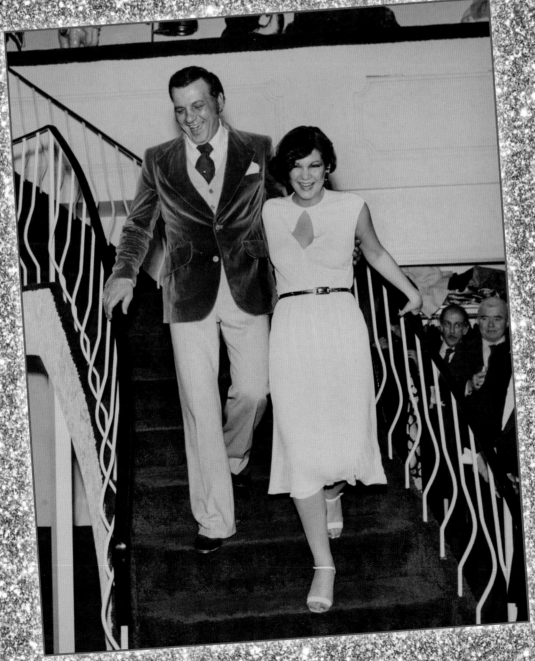

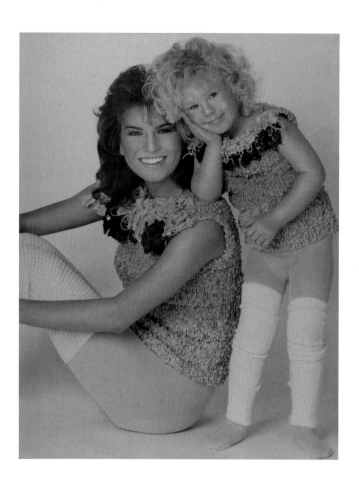

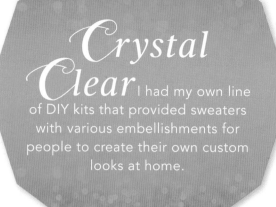
I was thrilled that my designs were selling and that my business was doing well. It felt great to get paid for something I loved doing. As I was growing up, Mom always used to say, "You have to work anyway, so why not find something you are passionate about and you will never be unhappy." Great advice, Mom!

My life was my work and my work was my life. It was always a dream of mine to run my own company. So, I spent my days designing embellished sweaters with big shoulder pads (very "in" at the time), while my nights were spent planning my own business. Finally, in 1981, I established the Sondra Celli Company by hand-knitting a custom line of children's outfits for boys and girls. My girls' line featured colorful ribbons, handmade flowers, and other embellishments, while my boys' line boasted adornments such as real checkers and tiny toy cars. I chose to create a children's line rather than pursue menswear because it took less capital to start up the business. For children's wear I needed only a small amount of yarn to make six knit samples, which I then marketed to wholesalers in New York. It took no time to find a sales representative to promote me. She booked me into a few trade shows where I could get exposure for my new line, and soon the orders began pouring in.

My line was picked up and sold in major department stores such as Bergdorf Goodman and Bloomingdales, as well as in several specialty shops across the country. To

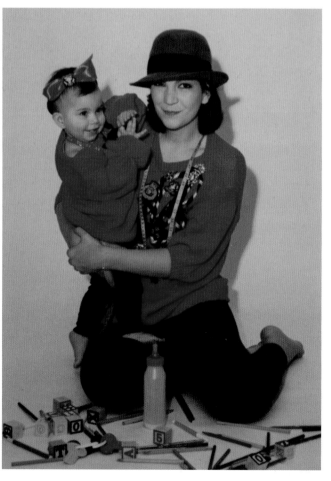

Above My sister, Linda, models a textured sweater from my first hand-knit collection. The line was created by using recycled jeans and assorted fabric remnants. 1980. *Courtesy of Sondra Celli*

Left My daughter, Milan, and I wearing matching knit designs from my line embellished with soutache and bouillon braid, tassels, and jewelry parts. 1990. *Courtesy of Sondra Celli*

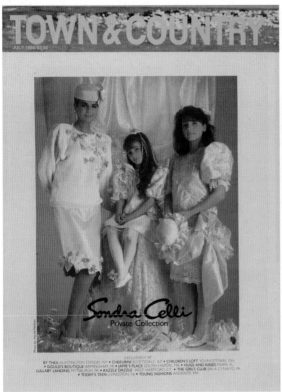

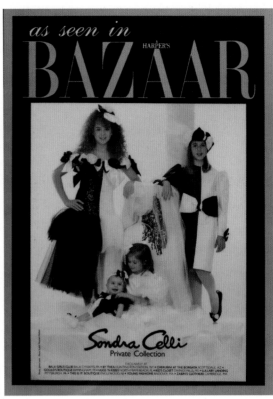

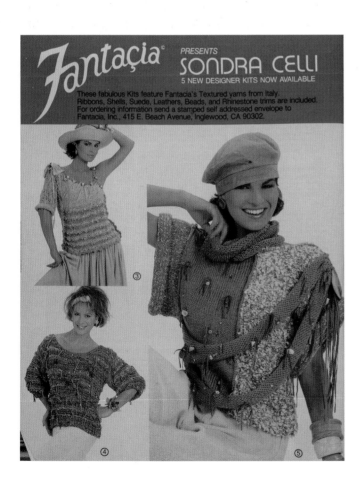

grow my business further, I applied to a program offering small businesses the opportunity to market to Asia. I was accepted and flew overseas to promote my designs. My line sold very well in Japan for many years. The market was particularly fond of my custom flower girl dresses.

As my business grew, I started traveling more, holding trunk shows in boutiques all over the United States to promote my children's line. I was still a solo act, designing, sewing, embellishing, and packing and shipping to department stores all over the country. I was the head designer, pattern maker, pattern cutter, seamstress, accountant, sales manager, publicist, marketing manager, inventory and quality control director, shipper, receptionist, receiver, and janitor. Anything that happened from the time I opened in the morning until I closed down at night was accomplished by a team of three–me, myself, and I.

Above My knitwear designs were featured in several publications, including *Town & Country*, *Harper's Bazaar*, and *Vogue*. 1988. *Courtesy of Sondra Celli*

Left Ad for Sondra Celli Designer Kits, presented by Fantaçia. 1982. *Courtesy of Sondra Celli*

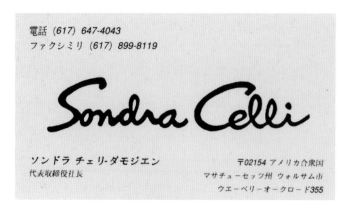

電話 (617) 647-4043
ファクシミリ (617) 899-8119

Sondra Celli

ソンドラ チェリ-ダモジエン
代表取締役社長

〒02154 アメリカ合衆国
マサチューセッツ州 ウォルサム市
ウエーベリーオークロード355

My Japanese business card, 1992. *Courtesy of Sondra Celli*

Opposite My children's knitwear line featured colorful, textural, and whimsical embellishments. I used mini race cars, tiny dinosaurs, assorted game pieces, and puffy paint. 1981. *Courtesy of Mark Johnson*

Working as an independent designer in New York City was tough, but I absolutely loved what I was doing. I remember sleeping on my work table at night in my clothes for an hour or two. That's all the time I could afford because there was so much to do. Thankfully, that all changed when Margie joined me.

Margie, a former coworker of mine and a recent retiree, knew of my overworked plight and offered to help. What an angel! Margie would hop a ride into the city with her husband, Frank, a meat packer. At four o'clock every morning, Frank would drop Margie off at my apartment and, after his shift, come by and pick her up to take her home. The first thing Margie did was make breakfast for me. Her maternal instincts ensured that I would have at least one hearty meal a day if she had anything to say about it. And oftentimes, after Margie left for the day, I would find a few beautiful steaks left covertly behind in my fridge. For six years I had the benefit of Margie's friendship and strong work ethic to help me get my business off the ground. Without Margie and Frank's help, I might never have made it in this business, and I certainly would not have eaten as well.

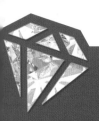

Crystal Clear

During the early days of starting my own business, I remember receiving a huge rush order on sweaters from a very high-end department store. Because the deadline was so tight, I decided to hire a freelance contractor. I shipped the sweater pieces off to her so that she would sew them together while I moved ahead on my other orders. When the box returned, I opened it up to check the work. To my horror, the first sweater had a tiny neck opening barely able to fit a Chihuahua, and certainly not a child. I pulled out another sweater, hoping the first one was just an aberration. It wasn't. The entire job was a disaster. For the next 24 hours straight, I feverishly ripped apart every sweater and then stitched them back together with a properly sized neck opening. When I finished the repair job I was utterly exhausted, but I made my deadline. Lesson learned? When you run a business, don't accept defeat. Do everything and anything you can to get the job done. You cannot afford to lose a sale or to let down a client.

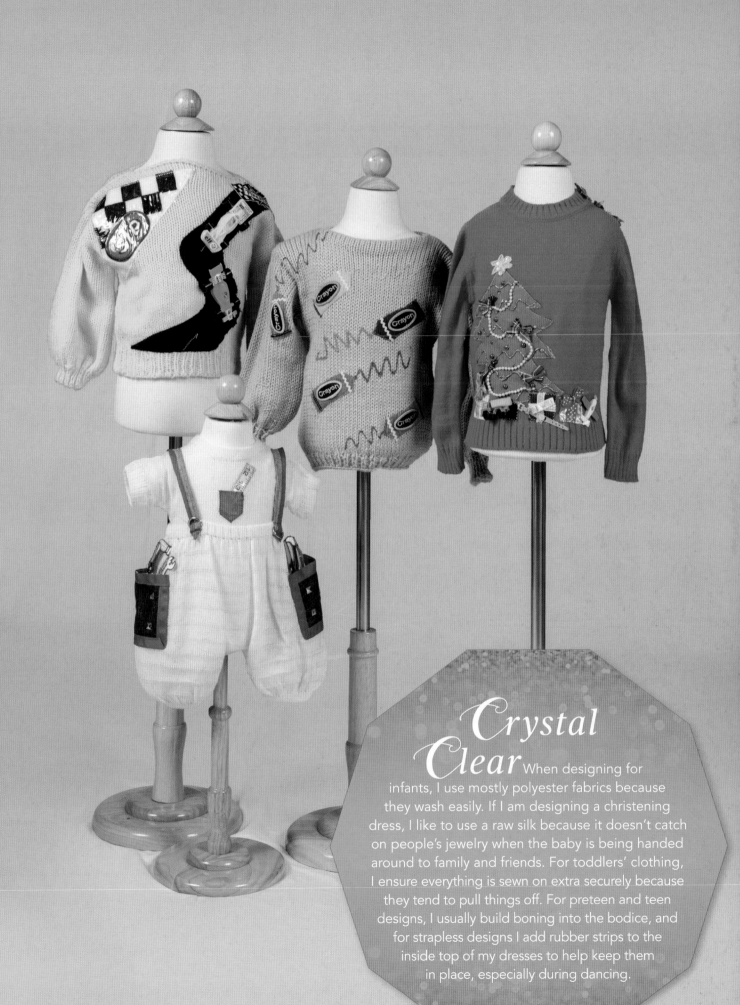

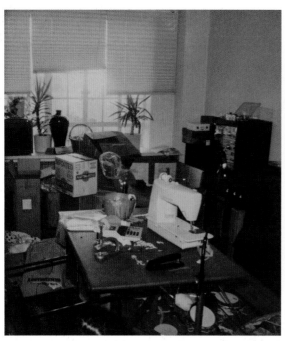

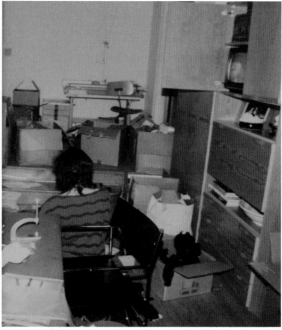

Eventually I moved my business into a loft on 38th Street, where I hired a few employees and sold to more department stores. I also transitioned into creating high-end custom clothing embellished with crystals. Crystals were coming into fashion at the time, and more and more customers were asking for them–both my Gypsy and non-Gypsy clients. As a designer, one is constantly innovating and must be on top of–or creating–the latest trends to stay relevant. In addition, working with crystals would be a new way to add value to my designs, allowing me to cut back on the number of pieces I would have to produce to make a living.

I was in that loft location for five years. In 1989, I became a mom to my beautiful daughter, Milan, named after my favorite city of fashion. Milan was looked after by a nanny, who would bring her to visit me at my work on a daily basis. When Milan was old enough, I would have her "help" me with little jobs or would give her fun art projects to keep her entertained. After a year or two of this, I decided on a major life change. I would leave New York to relocate my business back home to Boston.

I moved the Sondra Celli Company to Waltham, Massachusetts, in 1993 and set up shop in my mother's store. The main reason for returning home to the Boston area was to have the support of family while raising Milan and running my company.

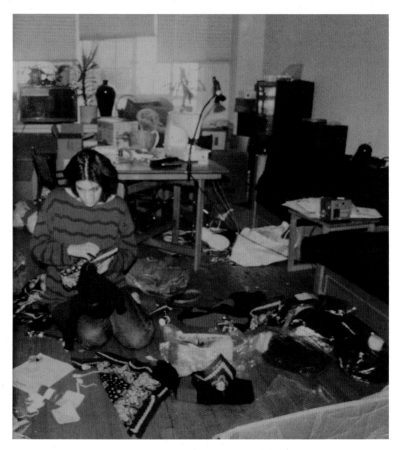

It may look cluttered to the untrained eye, but I see it as creativity at work. *Courtesy of Sondra Celli*

Above left When I decided to establish myself as an independent designer, I set up shop in my tiny 800-square-foot apartment. *Courtesy of Sondra Celli*

Above right Check out the "shipping department" for my budding business, 1989. *Courtesy of Sondra Celli*

I did well at Yolanda's. I had my own corner of the store where I displayed my bling-embellished children's line, which fit right in with my mom's glittering inventory. At the same time, I was able to help my mother by custom designing gowns, costumes, and props for her many fashion shows, fundraisers, and special events.

In 2010, I finally opened my own shop of "uncommon crystal couture," which now included designs for infants, preteens, teens, and adults featuring Swarovski® crystal embellishments. I moved into a historic redbrick building that was once the counting house for the Boston Manufacturing Company, a large cotton textile mill established in 1813. It is in a lovely location set alongside the Charles River. My inside space includes a small office plus two large, open rooms: a showroom and workroom. The exterior of my shop sports a blinged-out doorbell and crystal-packed sign designating my street address.

Right Milan, my best and most beautiful creation ever! 1989. *Courtesy of Sondra Celli*

Below left Nap time in a hatbox, 1993. *Courtesy of Sondra Celli*

Below right Milan "helps" with a design, 1996. *Courtesy of Sondra Celli*

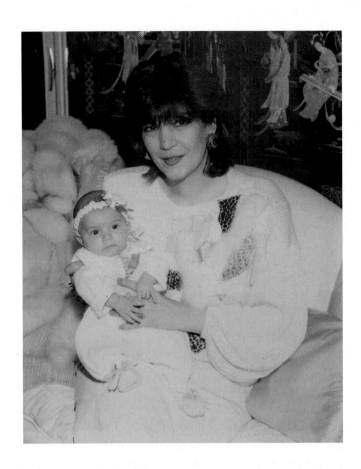

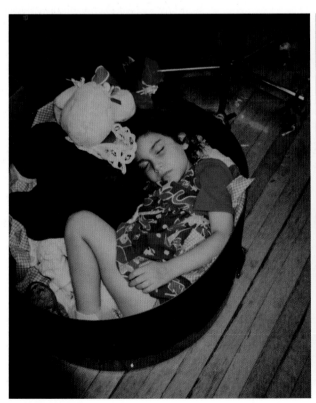

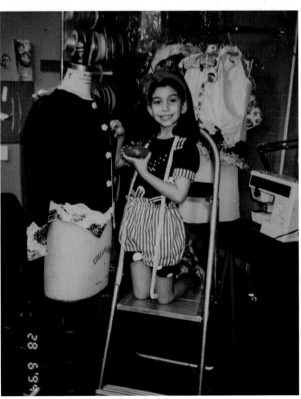

Crystal Clear

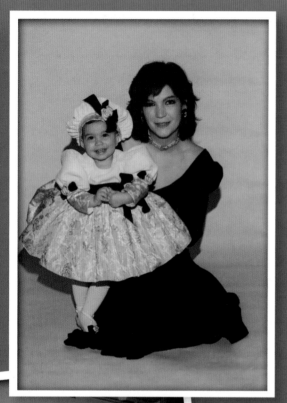

One of the many events I produced to promote my line was held seasonally at the Ritz Carlton Hotel in Boston. "Take Your Daughter to Lunch at the Ritz" would sell out every year. Informal modeling was done by the children of some of my clients. The kids loved being the center of attention in the sparkling party dresses and special occasion outfits, all festively embellished. It was rare that my inventory lasted through the afternoon, because most of the parents purchased the designs that their children modeled at the event. Naturally, Santa made an appearance at Christmastime, and, true to form, my Santa was elaborately clad in a custom gold suit I designed just for the occasion.

Top Milan in a custom Christmas dress I made, 1990.
Courtesy of Sondra Celli

Bottom left Milan with Santa in his glitzy suit, 1994.
Courtesy of Sondra Celli

Below "Take Your Daughter to Lunch at the Ritz" invitation.
Courtesy of Mark Johnson

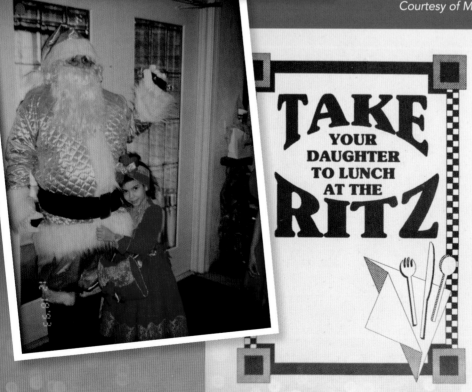

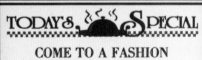

TODAY'S SPECIAL

COME TO A FASHION
SHOWING BY

Sondra Celli

OF 4–14 & PRETEEN
DRESSES & SUITS
FOR YOUR MOST
SPECIAL OCCASION
ON MARCH 19TH
12:00–3:00
R.S.V.P
Reservations for the
Ritz Carlton
dining room can be made
by calling 536-5700

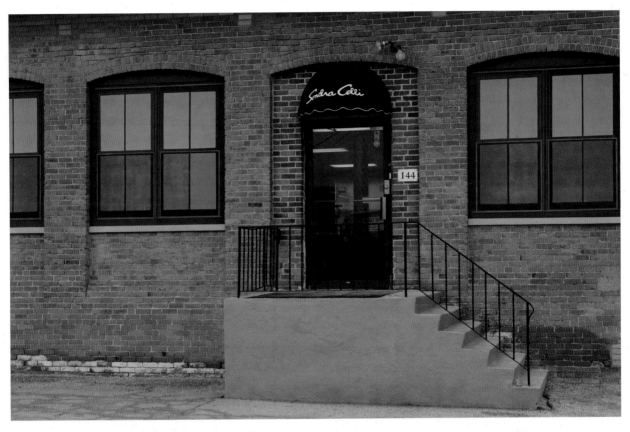

My shop is located about thirty minutes outside Boston in a historic red brick building. *Courtesy of Mark Johnson*

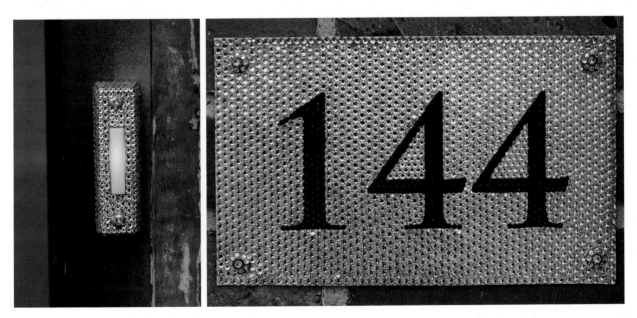

You can't miss my doorbell and address sign!
Courtesy of Mark Johnson

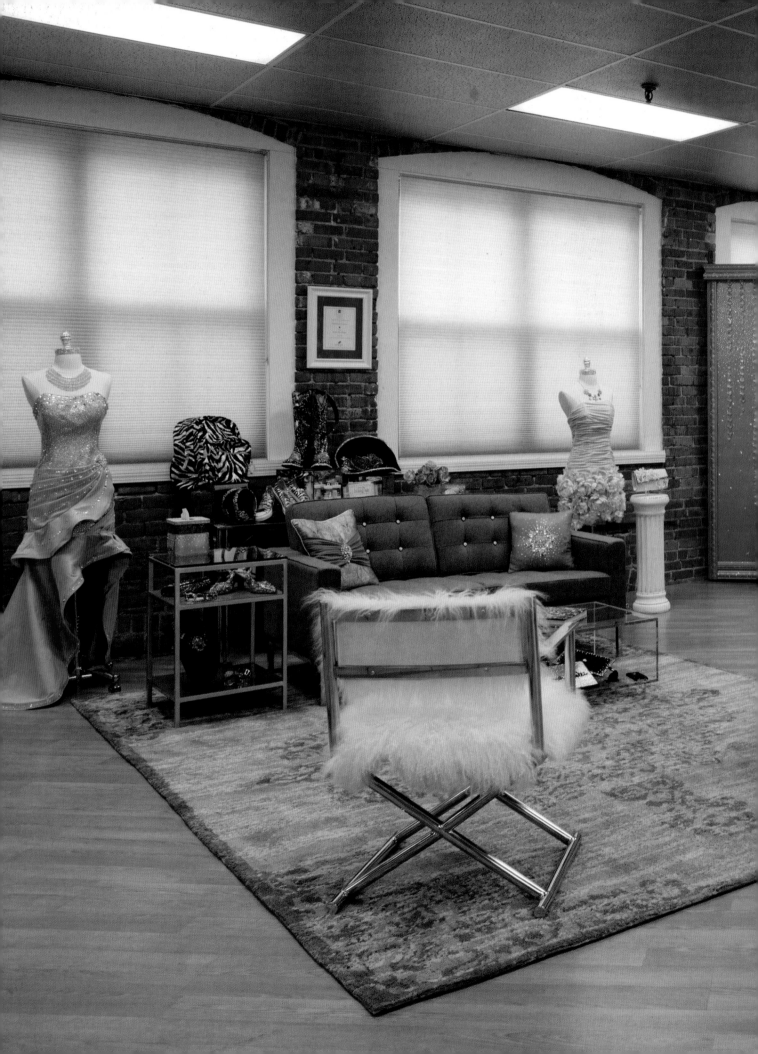

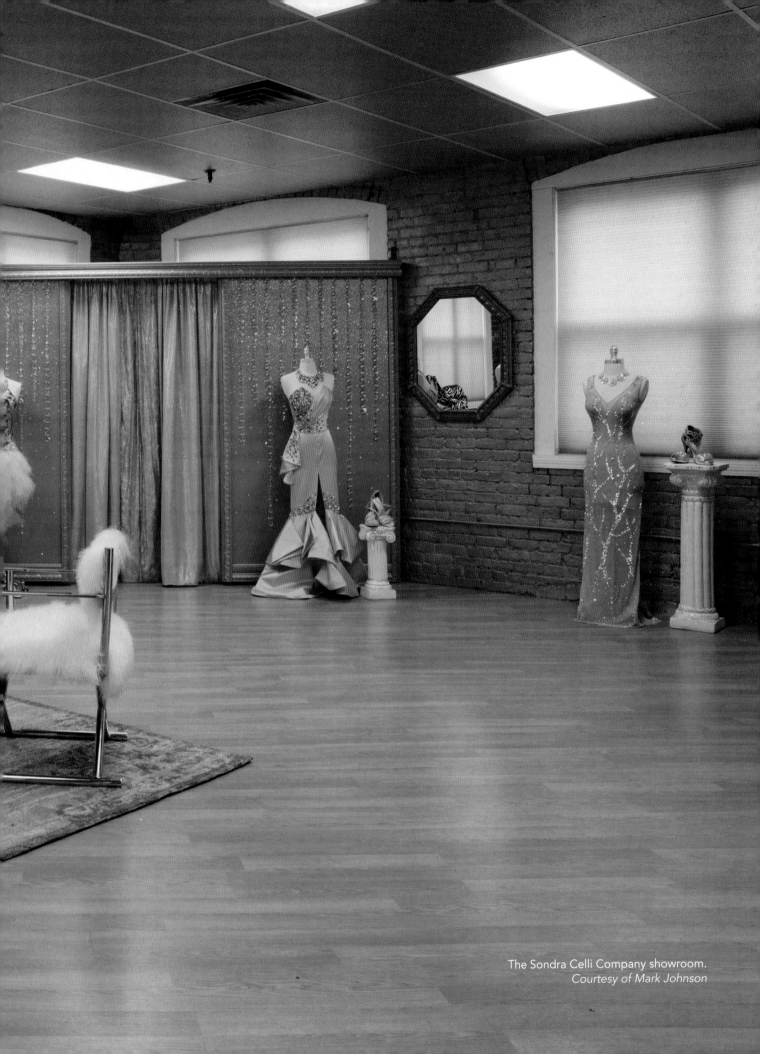

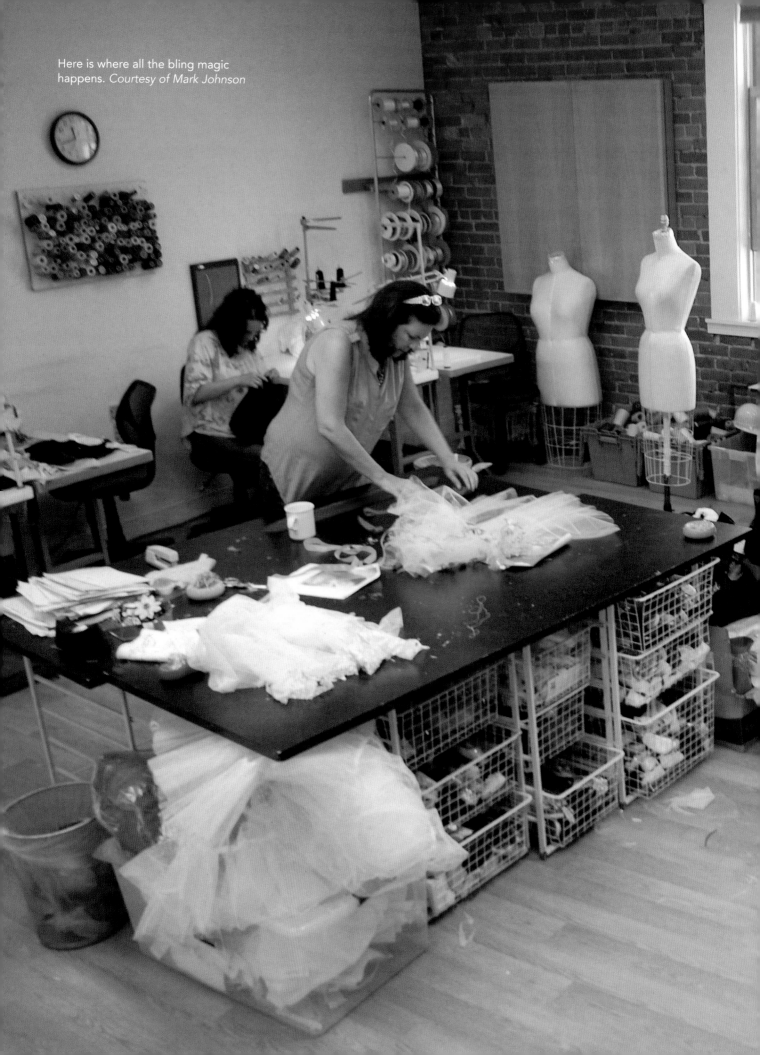

Here is where all the bling magic happens. *Courtesy of Mark Johnson*

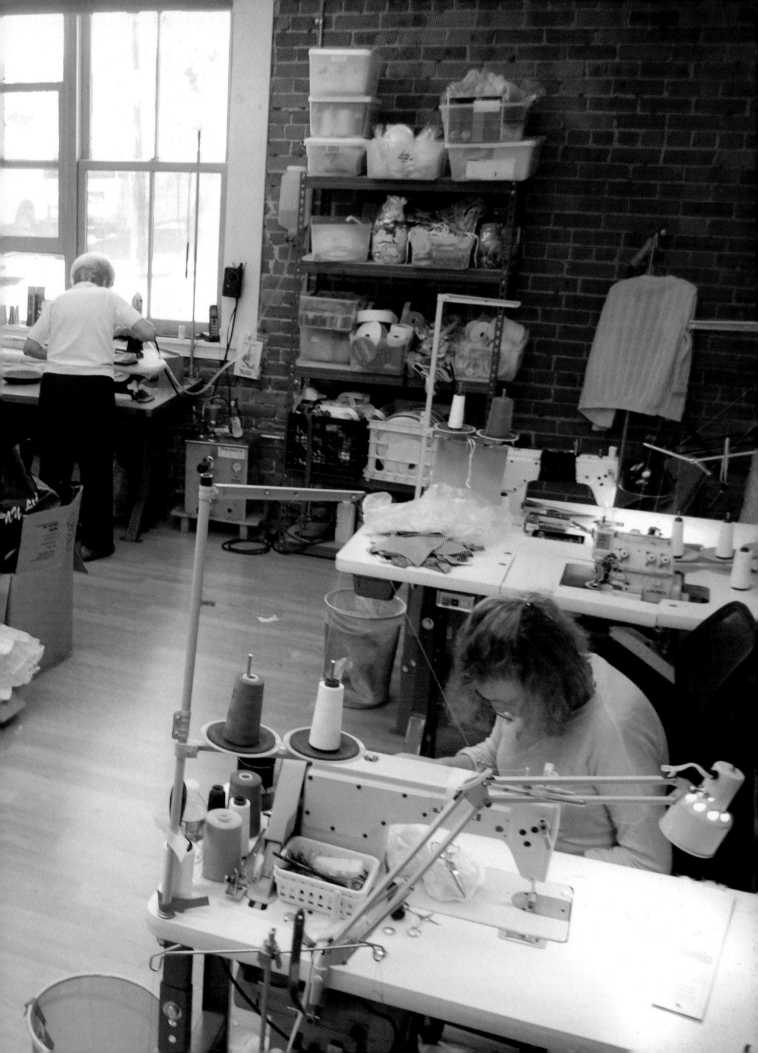

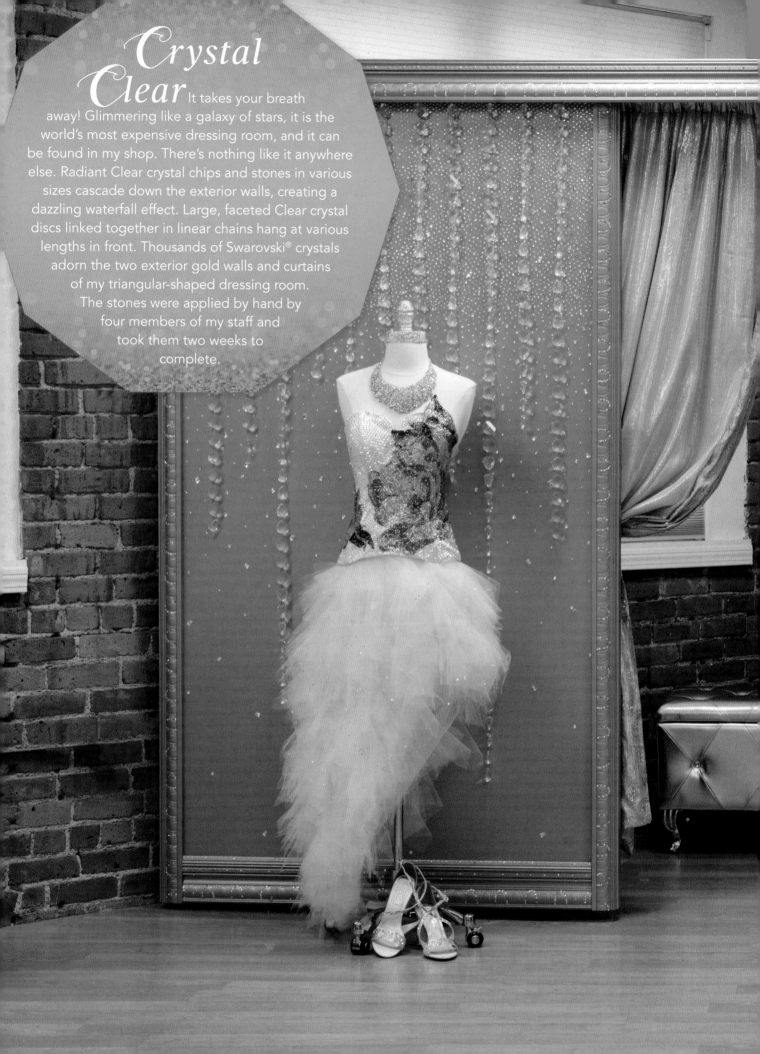

Crystal Clear

It takes your breath away! Glimmering like a galaxy of stars, it is the world's most expensive dressing room, and it can be found in my shop. There's nothing like it anywhere else. Radiant Clear crystal chips and stones in various sizes cascade down the exterior walls, creating a dazzling waterfall effect. Large, faceted Clear crystal discs linked together in linear chains hang at various lengths in front. Thousands of Swarovski® crystals adorn the two exterior gold walls and curtains of my triangular-shaped dressing room. The stones were applied by hand by four members of my staff and took them two weeks to complete.

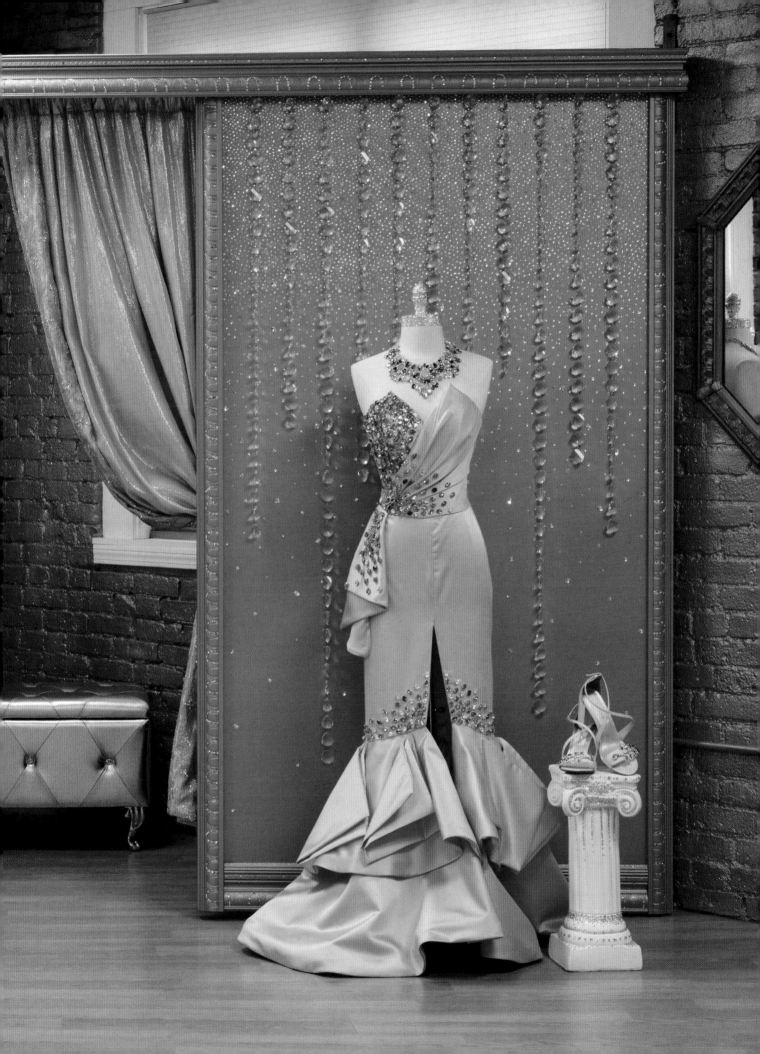

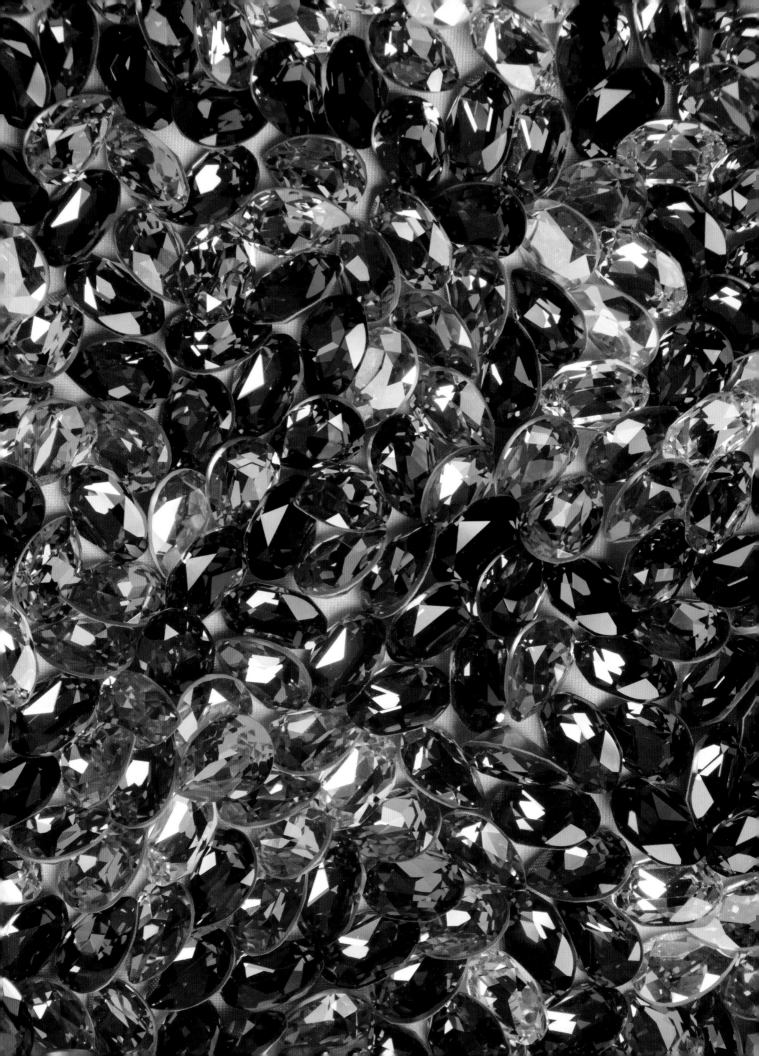

3.
Business of Bling

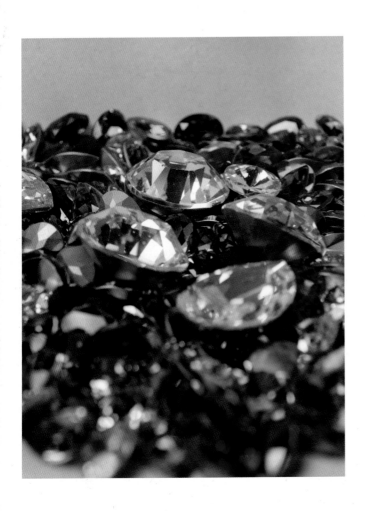

When it comes to bling, there's nothing like Swarovski®!
Courtesy of Mark Johnson

O n an average day I get to my shop at 6 a.m. and usually close by 6 p.m., unless we have a packed production schedule, and then I close later or sometimes pull an all-nighter. We make over 1,000 original custom creations annually, and some months are busier than others. For example, January is usually slow, while February begins the start of the busy bridal season. Prom orders start pouring in around March, and first-communion orders hit us about April, along with special outfits for prom and graduation. July can be quiet but we pick up steam again with numerous bat mitzvah orders in August. September keeps us busy with custom Halloween costume orders, and a lot of Gypsy parties are held in the fall calling for special bling outfits and accessories. In October, November, and December, we are as busy as Santa's elves, designing sparkly ensembles for the holiday season and New Year's festivities. Scattered throughout the entire year, orders come in for baby layettes, beauty pageant gowns, ballroom dance outfits, and a wide variety of other designs.

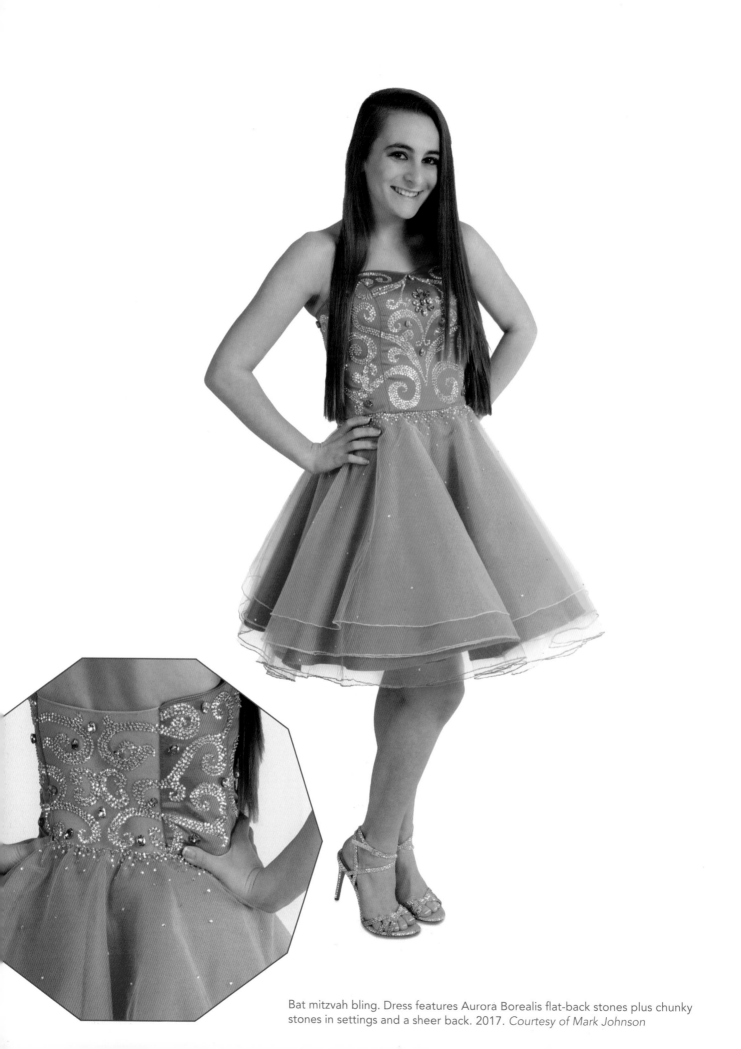

Bat mitzvah bling. Dress features Aurora Borealis flat-back stones plus chunky stones in settings and a sheer back. 2017. *Courtesy of Mark Johnson*

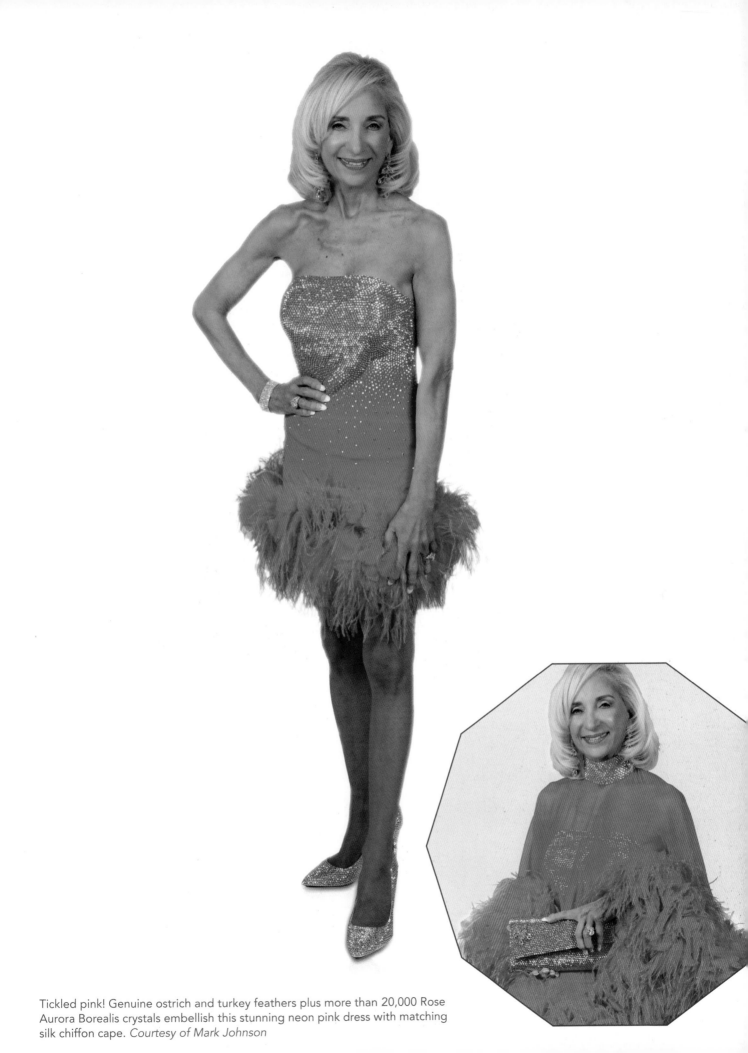

Tickled pink! Genuine ostrich and turkey feathers plus more than 20,000 Rose Aurora Borealis crystals embellish this stunning neon pink dress with matching silk chiffon cape. *Courtesy of Mark Johnson*

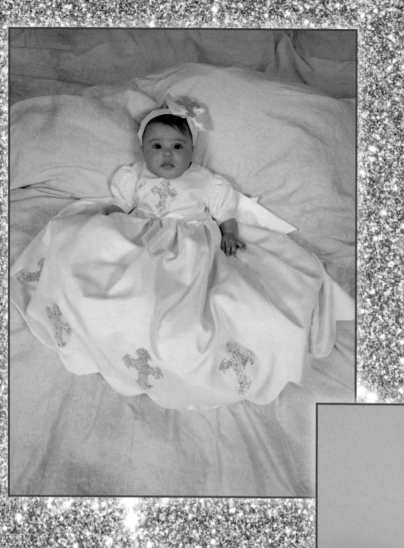

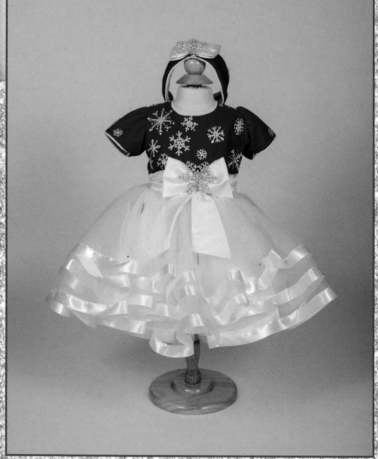

Baptism bling for baby. (Try saying that three times fast!) *Courtesy of Mark Johnson*

Baby's First Christmas dress, with sparkling snowflakes. *Courtesy of Mark Johnson*

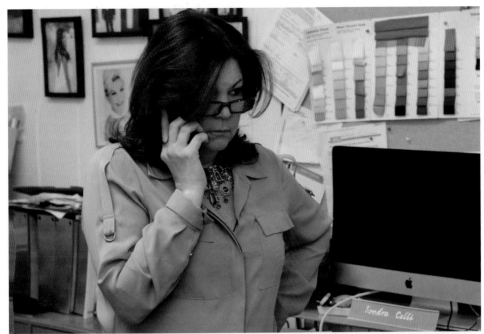

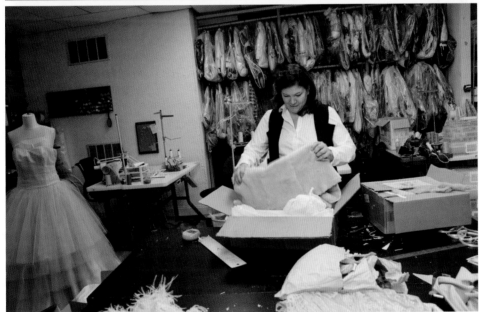

To run a successful business, it pays to be well organized, extremely flexible, and quick thinking. It's my job to ensure that my staff has all the stock they will need to complete every custom design on our production schedule, and that they are assigned the exact orders that we need to finish by the end of each work day.

In the workroom my responsibilities are to ensure that the sewing machines function properly, that scissors are sharp, and that the correct fabric, trim, thread, and zippers are on hand for every order, as well as the appropriate color, size, and number of crystals. I can't afford to have work stop because a machine is down or we have run out of stones.

I order in all the fabrics and embellishments for every custom design made by my staff. I am constantly tracking which supplies are being delivered and whether they will arrive in the morning or afternoon, so that my staff isn't kept waiting for supplies they need to begin their work day. Organization is the key to productivity.

Top On the phone from the time I wake up until I fall asleep—hopefully by 10 p.m. *Courtesy of Mark Johnson*

Bottom When supplies arrive on time it's a very good day. *Courtesy of Mark Johnson*

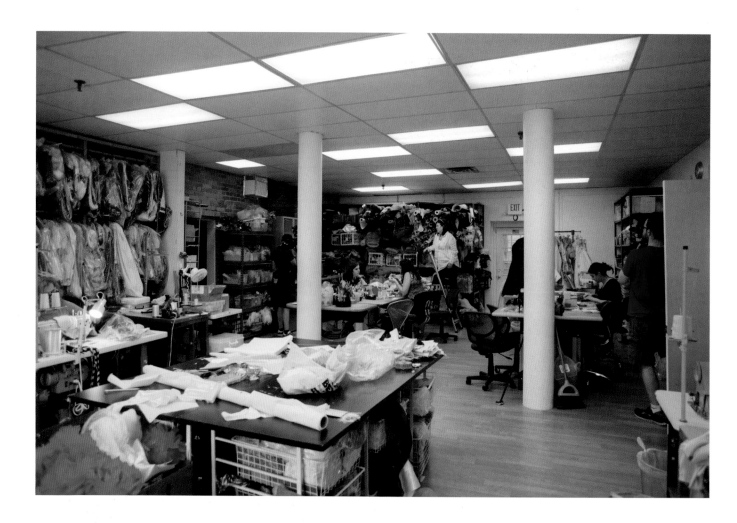

Flexibility and quick thinking come when there is a packed schedule to contend with. We run a tight ship, and each member of the Sondra Celli team is integral to getting creations out the door on time. If one of my staff calls in sick, my entire schedule gets flipped around and I must quickly rethink the calendar and production schedule to see how that absent person's projects will get done. Or, perhaps a bride calls to have her dress finished earlier or a client changes her mind on a design or a snowstorm delays a shipment of materials. Work can't grind to a halt when there's a bit of a hiccup. I just have to review the situation and come up with a different plan.

My work schedule can also be affected when someone unexpectedly shows up at the door. Although we are an appointment-only shop, there are times when the doorbell rings and a fan or potential client will be standing at the door. I merely rework my schedule to fit them in. As a business owner, I never turn away a potential client, and, as a TV personality, I would never turn away fans who have traveled miles to meet me. *My Big Fat American Gypsy Wedding* airs internationally, so it's not unusual to have folks from all over the globe drop in while they are vacationing in the area. For anyone who has traveled a long distance just to meet me, I figure the least I can do is take time out to visit. And if they are kind enough to call ahead to let me know they are coming, I make sure to have one of my homemade cheesecakes ready for them.

Above It's always a busy workroom. *Courtesy of Mark Johnson*

Opposite top Surprise visits from fans happen most often in the summer. *Courtesy of Mark Johnson*

Opposite bottom Whenever I make a cheesecake, it always comes embellished. *Courtesy of Mark Johnson*

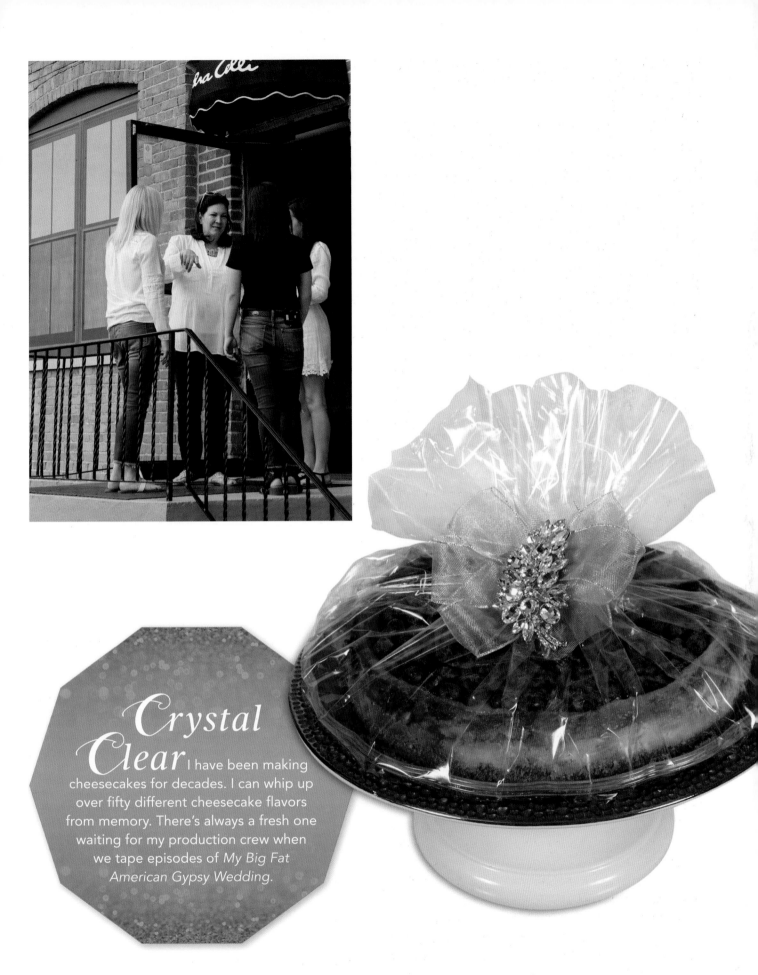

Crystal Clear

I have been making cheesecakes for decades. I can whip up over fifty different cheesecake flavors from memory. There's always a fresh one waiting for my production crew when we tape episodes of *My Big Fat American Gypsy Wedding*.

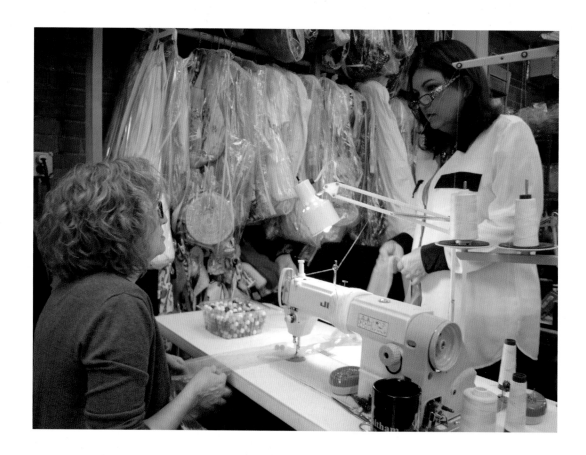

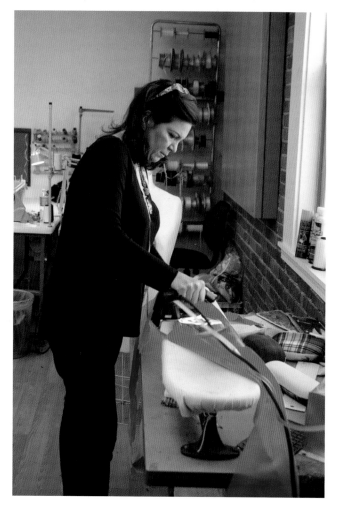

Above Mira sews gumballs into the hem of a candy dress we designed for the show. *Courtesy of Mark Johnson*

Left Believe it or not, I find ironing relaxing. *Courtesy of Mark Johnson*

Opposite top Farrah uses the bling tool to stone a pair of heels. *Courtesy of Tisi Farrar*

Opposite bottom Discussing design layout. *Courtesy of Mark Johnson*

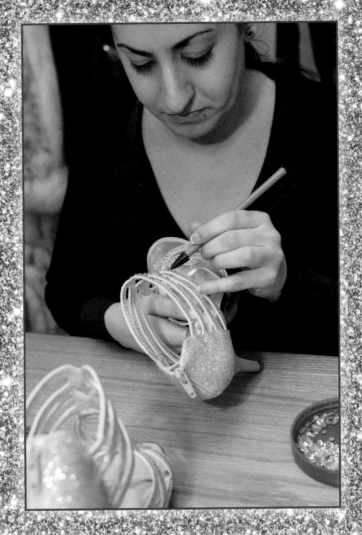

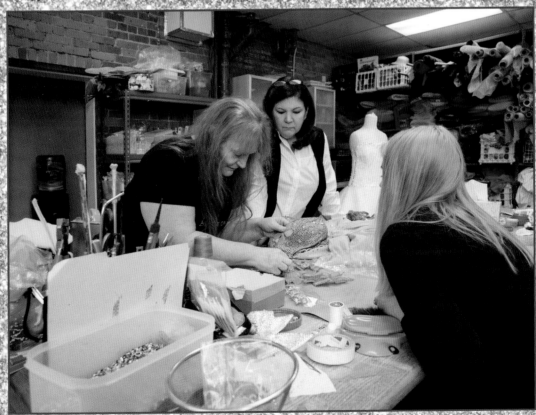

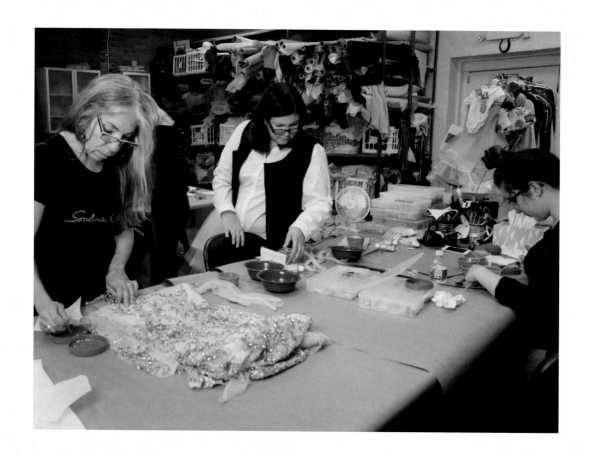

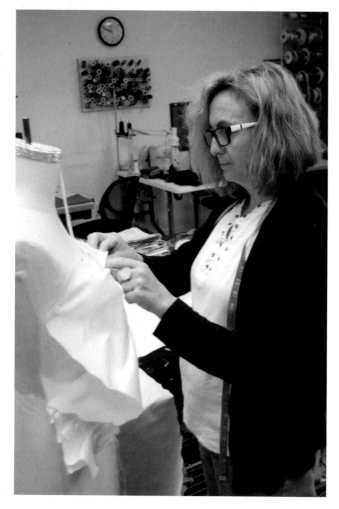

Above and left *Courtesy of Mark Johnson*

Opposite top For quinceañeras we create a custom dress for the celebrant as well as an exact copy of the dress for the "Last Doll." The doll signifies a young girl's transition from childhood into womanhood (symbolized by storing away her last doll). *Courtesy of Mark Johnson*

Opposite bottom This corset is embellished with jewelry pieces, and then individual stones are added in a tight dot pack motif to fill up the bodice. *Courtesy of Tisi Farrar*

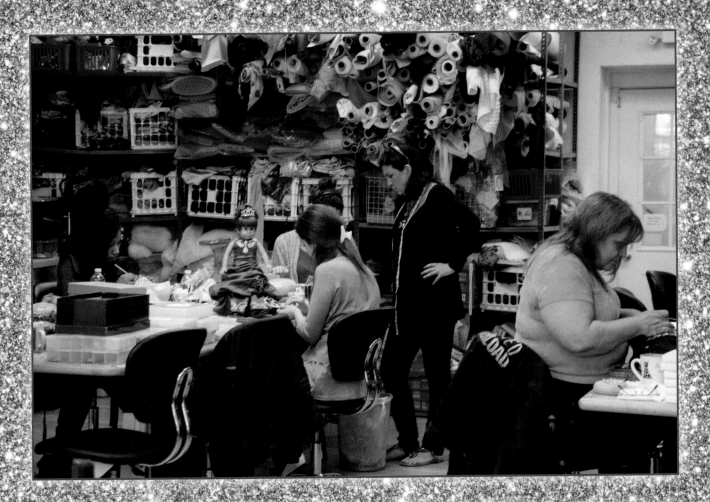
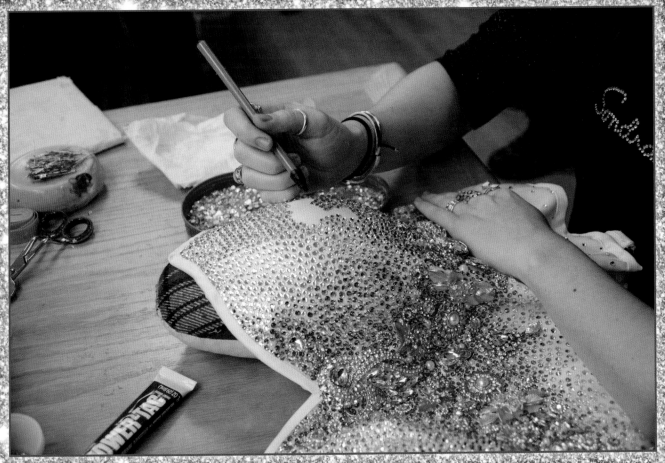

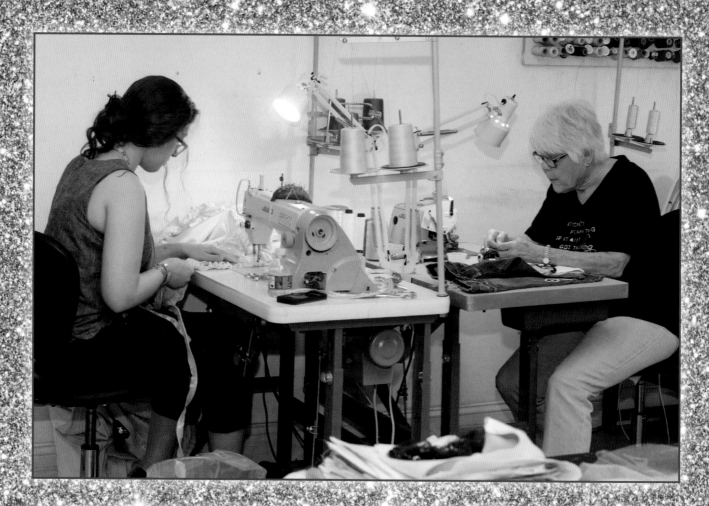

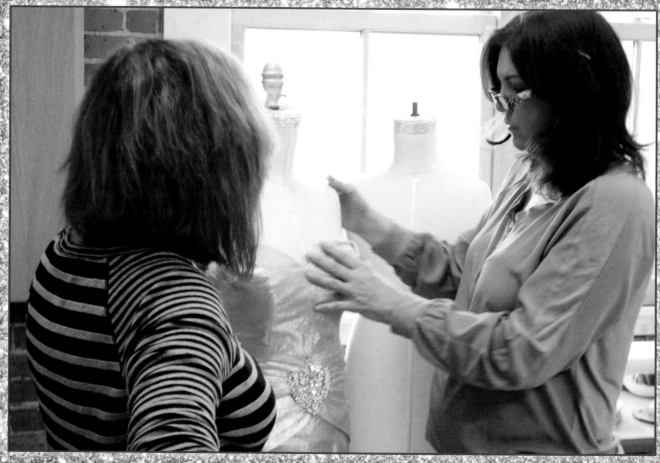

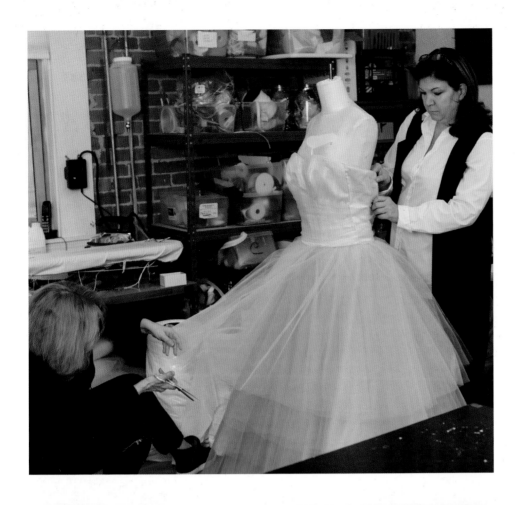

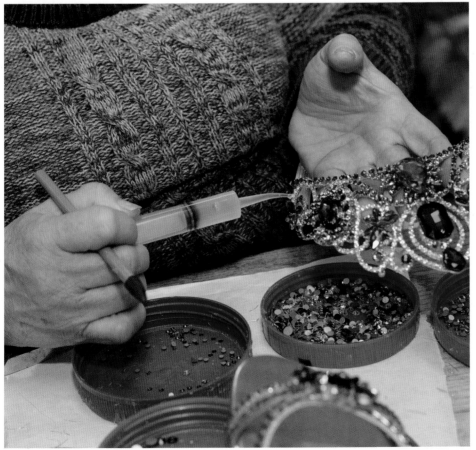

Opposite top Amelia sews up a skirt while Diane separates stones into color and size categories. *Courtesy of Mark Johnson*

Opposite bottom Mira and I are constantly brainstorming ideas as the designs evolve. *Courtesy of Mark Johnson*

Above *Courtesy of Mark Johnson*

Left Carol applies additional stones to a tiara for added brilliance. Using a bling tool to pick up crystals saves time, especially when doing intricate stonework. *Courtesy of Mark Johnson*

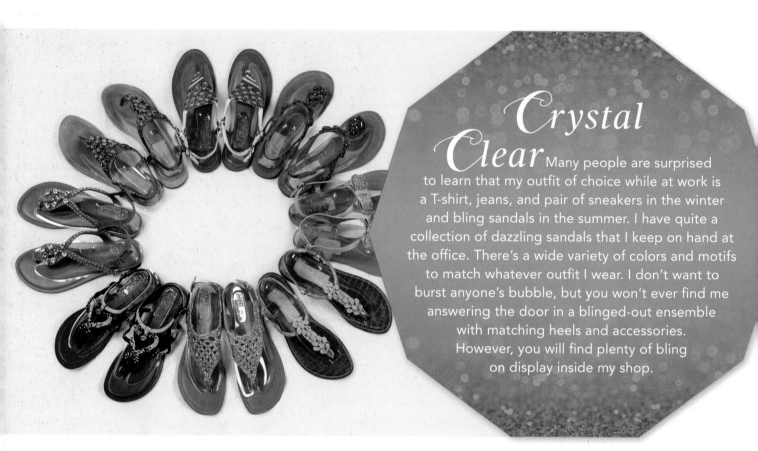

Crystal Clear

Many people are surprised to learn that my outfit of choice while at work is a T-shirt, jeans, and pair of sneakers in the winter and bling sandals in the summer. I have quite a collection of dazzling sandals that I keep on hand at the office. There's a wide variety of colors and motifs to match whatever outfit I wear. I don't want to burst anyone's bubble, but you won't ever find me answering the door in a blinged-out ensemble with matching heels and accessories. However, you will find plenty of bling on display inside my shop.

I move from office to showroom to workroom and back again throughout the day, constantly multitasking. In my office I check voice mails, call vendors, order office supplies (as well as fabrics, trims, and crystals), respond to social media, open mail, handle correspondence, file, and pay bills. In the showroom I meet with clients, fans, and the media and, when we are in production, shoot episodes of the show. I also set up photo shoots, create new displays, and do much of the packing and shipping.

Seems like a really packed day, doesn't it? It gets even busier when the TV production crew shows up to record episodes for *My Big Fat American Gypsy Wedding*. They normally spend two consecutive days shooting at my shop every two weeks. During that time we work together, shooting the making of the dress to be featured on the show or my in-person meetings with

or phone calls to the Gypsy brides. Once the cameras are off, I go back to my "to do" list for the day. Somehow it all works.

When I initially began to focus on building my business around custom designs and accessories embellished with bling, it started slowly at first but then flourished. Sparkling accents grab your attention and can transform something drab into something brilliant. This is especially true when using Swarovski® crystals.

Above Enjoy extremely happy feet in a pair of bling sandals! *Courtesy of Mark Johnson*

Opposite Can you see the difference? In a matchup of plastic "crystals" (*left*) vs. Swarovski® (*right*), there is no contest. *Courtesy of Mark Johnson*

I oversee and direct every design project that my staff is working on, and know exactly how long it will take them to finish each design, so that I can ensure every deadline is met. A large part of my day is spent cutting out patterns. Since I do most of the cutting for all the designs we make, I can sometimes stand at my worktable for hours. On the other end of the process, once a design is complete, I inspect it to ensure quality control, then tag it, pack it, address it, and ship it.

So how does the design process start? When a customer is interested in ordering a custom design, I first ask them to send me a photo or sketch of what they have in mind. If they don't have a visual or don't know exactly what they are looking for, I will offer suggestions. Once I have a visual starting point, it enables me to provide the client with a price estimate, and, if that price fits within their budget, we can proceed to discuss details such as specific fabrics, colors, amount of bling, and what, if any, matching accessories they might want. Then my staff and I get to work cutting, sewing, and embellishing to make people's dreams come true. The amount of time it takes to create a design is based on the style and how busy we are at the time that the order is placed. A wedding dress can take anywhere from two to six months, while a baby's first-birthday dress can take a week.

Crystal Clear

Back in 1895, Daniel Swarovski designed an innovative machine capable of cutting crystals more precisely than by hand. His dream was to create "a diamond for everyone." Today, Swarovski® is world renowned for producing the finest crystals, boasting unparalleled clarity in vibrant colors. That is why Swarovski® has such a global following. Their sparkling decorations have dominated in the worlds of fashion, art, design, décor, theater, and film for decades. Why do I prefer Swarovski®? They provide an unmatched quality of sparkle when light is refracted by the precision-cut multifaceted surfaces of the stones. Any ensemble or accessory embellished with these glittering stones jumps to life in tiny explosions of blazing color and shine, sparked by every move you make. Manufactured in Austria, they are the best of the best man-made crystals and, although expensive, worth the price, since you cannot find a more brilliant embellishment short of real diamonds.

Crystal Clear

If I am working with a client who loves sparkle but doesn't have a large budget, Czechoslovakian glass stones can often do the trick. Although they don't have as many facets as Swarovski® stones, they do provide a lovely glittering effect. I avoid plastic stones entirely. They lack brilliance and look cheap.

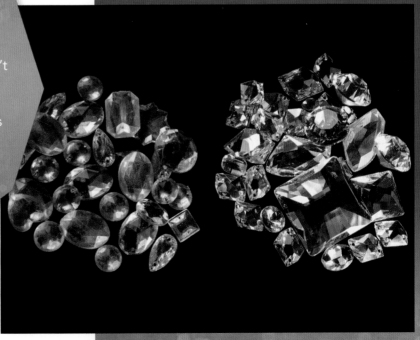

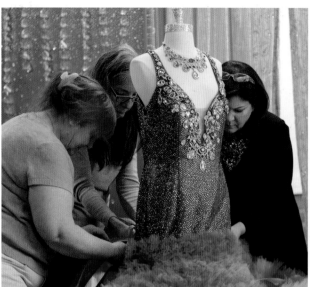 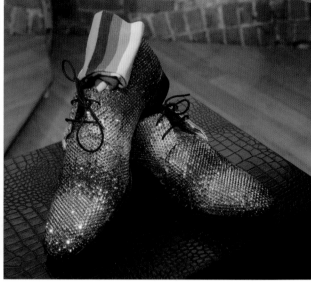

My Gypsy and Traveler clients love to pack their clothes with sparkling stones. It's like a competition for them. Whoever has the most stones wins. In their cultures, the more bling you can pack on, the louder your message. It's a way of visually communicating to others that you are well off and well cared for, as bling can be pricey! Centuries ago, Gypsies, who migrated from India, were constantly moving to avoid persecution. The Travelers, mostly of Irish descent, were also on the move fleeing prejudice. Both nomadic groups would carry all their worldly possessions with them as they roamed. Women wore their wealth, draping themselves with bangles, earrings, and necklaces. Today they still drape themselves, but with clothes and accessories packed with bling.

It's interesting to note that wearing one's wealth is also a common trait among the men of the Gypsy and Traveler communities. One of the most ornate designs I ever embellished was a man's jacket featuring a climbing vine motif packed with hundreds of thousands of crystals. It was quite impressive and must have made for a very dramatic entrance.

Left This satin dress was adorned with 300 multicolored jewels and 17,000 Tanzanite crystals. *Courtesy of Mark Johnson*

Right Even guys like bling. These rainbow ombré shoes boast 12,000 stones! *Courtesy of Mark Johnson*

Opposite top Yes, I do bling for pets. Sparkle, my Coton de Tulear, models a harness with matching leash blinged out in a zebra motif. *Courtesy of Mark Johnson*

Opposite bottom Sparkle in the custom Gypsy-style wedding dress I designed for her to wear in the 2017 Waltham Riverfest Pets on Parade competition. I am proud to say that she won first place and a best-dressed award. *Courtesy of Mark Johnson*

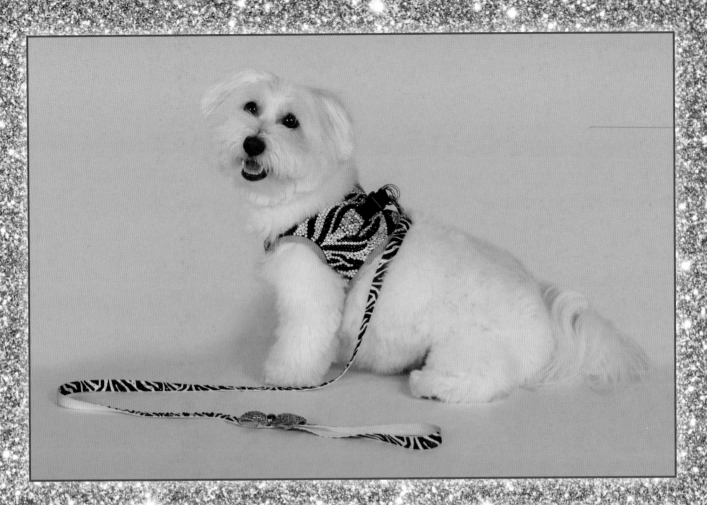
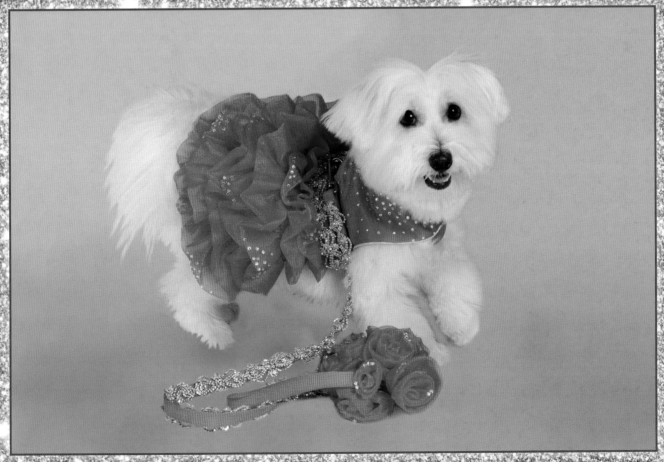

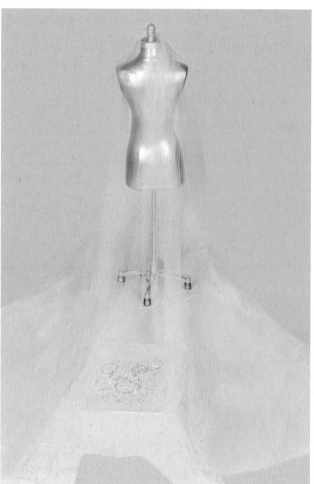

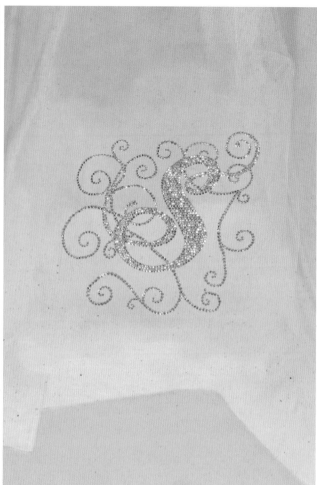

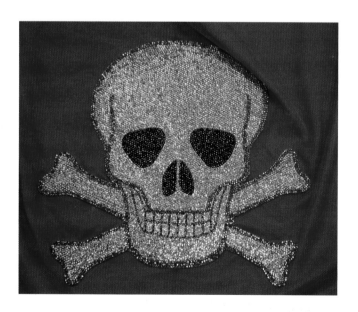

people wearing bling at all hours of the day and almost everywhere: on campus, in the gym, at the mall, grocery store, or vacation resort. Bling is a hot fashion trend and very much in demand.

At times we are asked by clients to embellish a dress, jacket, or pair of shoes that they already own but that looks too plain. We can easily transform these items into something special by adding bling. We have added "Happily Ever After," using stones to personalize a bride's store-bought veil, and designed intertwined hearts with the couple's initials on a bride's train. Crystal embellishments give life to any design. They are such attention-getting accents and I believe they make people happy. How can

Above Crystal-monogrammed wedding veil. *Courtesy of Mark Johnson*

Left We created this skull-and-crossbones motif on a dress train for a motorcycle-loving bride. *Courtesy of Tisi Farrar*

My non-Gypsy clients run the gamut from newborn to senior citizen and from cheerleader and pageant contestant to working mom and executive. You'll find

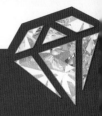

Crystal Clear

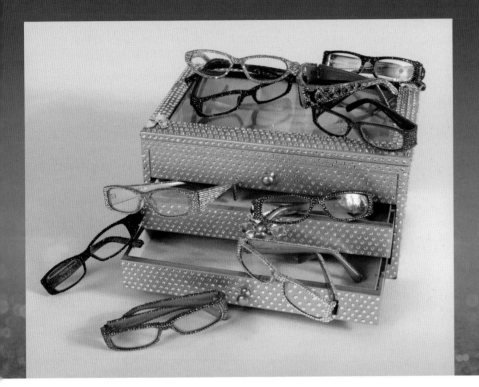

I usually suggest that clients purchase my bling glasses packed with Clear crystals. It is the actual name given to a Swarovski® stone that resembles ice. It has no color to it and therefore complements any colors it is matched with. We can also bling out personal prescription eyeglass frames if you ship them to us.

An assortment of sparkling specs.
Courtesy of Mark Johnson

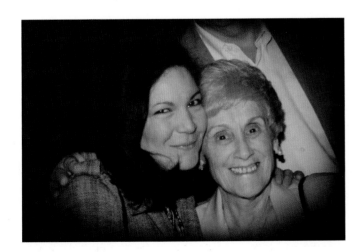

you be sad when your clothing is animated by flashes of light reflecting off multifaceted crystals?

Every project we create is unique. Our number-one-selling accessory is our custom bling eyeglasses. They are "cheaters" (or "readers") covered in crystals. If you watch *My Big Fat American Gypsy Wedding* then you have probably seen me wearing them. We bling them out in a wide variety of colors. You can also have a choice of motifs such as leopard, zebra, floral, polka dot, and ombré. The frames are packed by using three different sizes of stones. The smaller the stones, the more intricate and time-consuming the process, but the outcome is stunning.

My small staff consists of a talented group of veteran seamstresses and artistic designers (affectionately known as the "Bling-ettes") who do the crystal embellishment work. They work hard and can create any and every design I throw at them. They are like family and have been with me for quite a while. One woman, Jeanette, worked for me for twenty-four years and recently retired at the age of ninety-two!

Left Jeanette was my longest-serving employee and a real spitfire. *Courtesy of Sondra Celli*

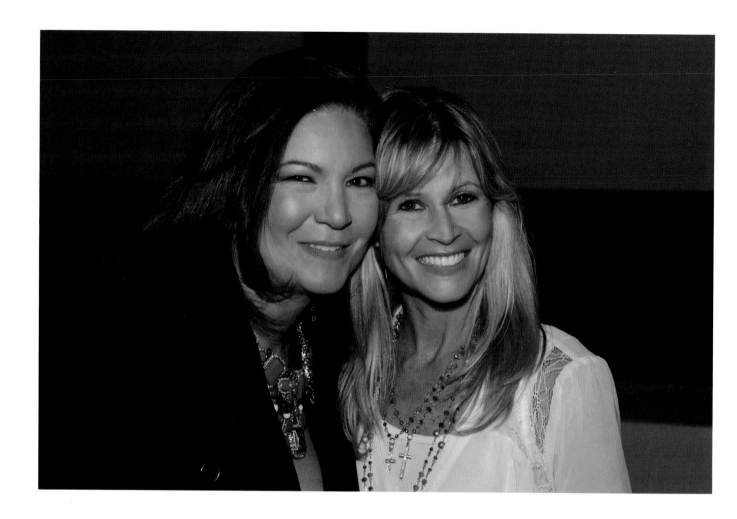

Most of the Bling-ettes have advanced design degrees. We train them on the various bling techniques when they join our staff. The three primary techniques are called Dot Pack, Interlock, and Pack-and-Fade. Starting with chapter 7, we provide instructions on each of those techniques so that you can learn how to "bling it on" at home.

In 2013, I received a call from Tracy Sormanti, director of the New England Patriots Cheerleaders (NEPC), who was looking for a designer to update her squad's look with a new uniform and bling. I was thrilled and asked her how she found me. Apparently, Tracy's neighbor was a huge fan of my work on *My Big Fat American Gypsy Wedding* and was emphatic that Tracy call me first. Thankfully, Tracy listened to her and I was hired.

The uniform features a top with long sheer sleeves and a pair of short shorts. I created a second halter top to coordinate with the shorts and added matching wrist bands. The uniform was embellished with Light Siam, Clear, and Crystal Metallic Blue crystals. Five New England Patriots logos adorn each uniform set. It was a time-consuming process, since the logos had to be hand-drawn first to provide a "map" for the Bling-ettes to follow when arranging the stones. A variety of seven sizes of stones were used. Each logo is made up of 2,400 stones, and more stones were used for trim work. To outfit the entire squad, roughly 600,000 crystals were used.

Whether the women are cheering on the five-time Super Bowl-winning New England Patriots under the afternoon sun or stadium lights, the bling-embellished uniforms infuse every kick and jump with an unparalleled luminescent energy. Designing for Tracy and her impressive squad of beautiful, phenomenally talented, and highly accomplished women is one of the highlights of my career.

Above New England Patriots Cheerleaders director extraordinaire, Tracy Sormanti. *Courtesy of Mark Johnson*

Opposite Two talented members of the New England Patriots Cheerleaders, Bailey and Isabella, wearing the custom bling uniforms I designed with NEPC director Tracy Sormanti. *Courtesy of Robert Hare*

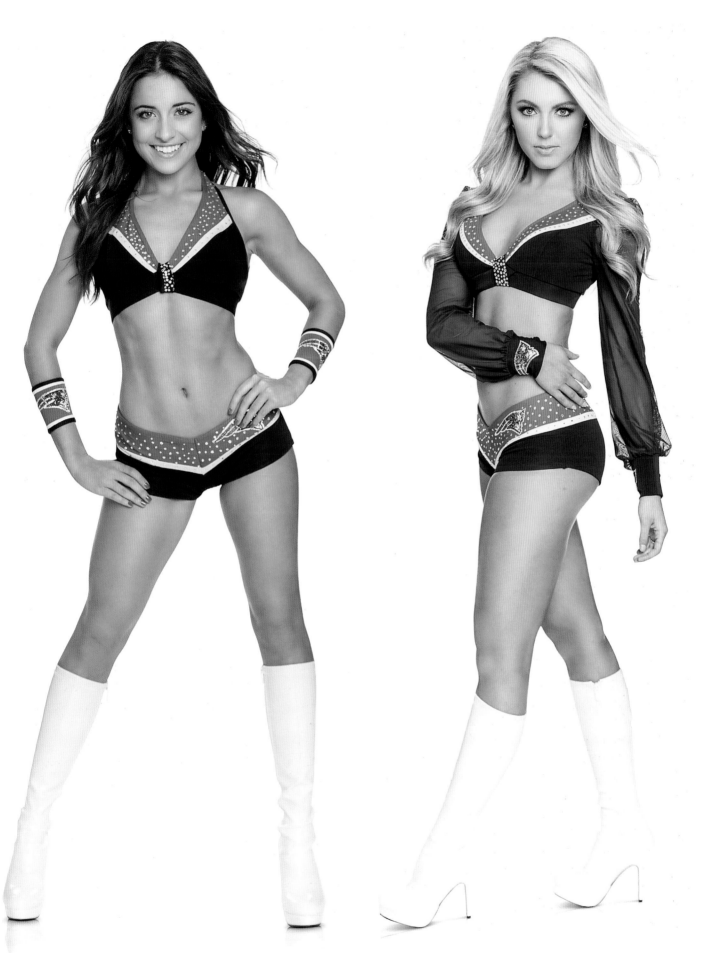

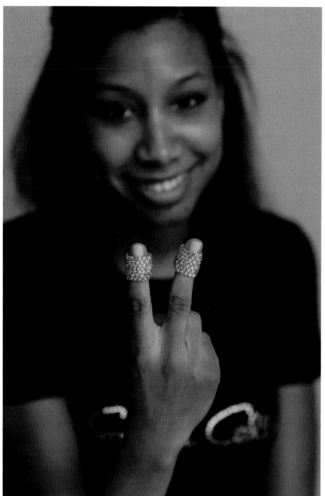

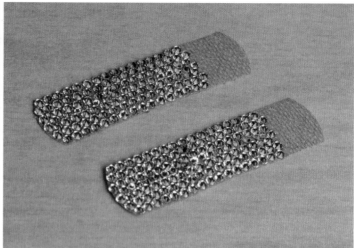

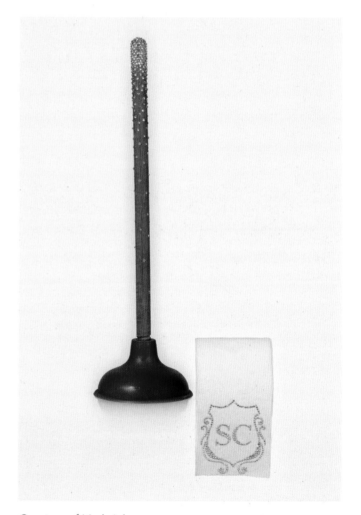

Courtesy of Mark Johnson

Some of the most unusual items we have been asked to bling include blades of a ceiling fan, pots and pans (for decorative purposes only), a basketball, bandages, a toilet plunger, and toilet paper. The blinged-out bandages were commissioned by a client who was attending a black-tie affair and had ordered a custom gown from us for the occasion. The day before her event, she called us in a panic because she had lost one of her manicured nails and didn't want an ugly bandage to ruin the appearance of her gown. We added stones that matched the color of her gown to two bandages (one to wear and one backup), and delivered them to her in time for her gala. She said the bling bandage was the main topic of interest all night long.

The custom-blinged toilet paper was ordered by another client who was holding an open house. She thought it would be fun to add a little sparkle to her home and asked that we create a crystal monogram to "dress up" the guest bathroom. (I told her if she wanted to flush her money down the toilet, it was OK with me.)

I think the only request we have turned down so far is to bling out the hubcaps of a car. The extreme changes of weather and temperature could affect the adhesive nature of the glue, and the driver could end up leaving a trail of sparkling stones in the dust.

For the most part, however, if it can sit still, we can bling it.

4.
Bling, Gypsies, Travelers, and Me

Everyone always wants to know how I started designing for the Gypsy and Traveler communities. It actually began more than thirty-five years ago when they found me.

I had a signature children's line that was being carried in several major department store chains across the country. It was a colorful line with fanciful embellishments and was selling well. One particular week I was bombarded with calls from a number of independent boutiques wanting to buy my line. I started taking orders and shipping boxes of my product to "Annie's Boutique," "Crystal's Boutique," "Bridgette's Boutique," and other similarly named shops. The strange thing was that every one of those shops was in the same city and had the same street address but a different number. I couldn't figure it out. How could so many boutiques stay in business if they were located right next door to one another? Not until I told a friend who was a veteran in the fashion industry about the strange coincidence did I get an explanation. She laughed and told me, "Honey, those aren't shops

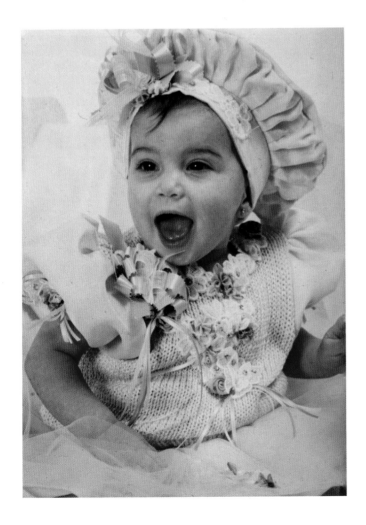

My daughter, Milan, in one of my early knitwear designs. Pieces from this line caught the eyes of the Gypsies; they loved the fanciful embellishments. 1989. *Courtesy of Sondra Celli*

55

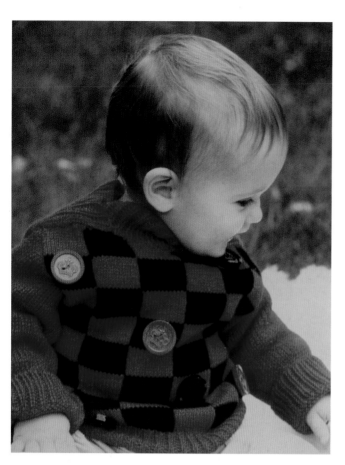

you are selling to; you're shipping to Irish Travelers living in the same neighborhood!" Apparently, one of the Travelers had convinced a sales clerk to hand over my contact number. Word travels fast in the Traveler community, and soon everyone was calling. From there, word spread among the Gypsy community and the phone rang 24/7!

At the time I really had no idea what a "Gypsy" was, but I quickly learned as my client base grew to include more and more Romanichal and Irish Traveler clients. It's been a rewarding experience. I am so grateful that after more than thirty-five years I am still the one they call when they want custom designs for special occasions.

Left This checkerboard sweater was a huge hit. It was the first of my designs to get placed into department stores. I bought all the checkers available at a local Woolworth's, drilled holes into them, and hand-stitched them onto sweaters. 1981. *Courtesy of Sondra Celli*

Below Gypsy baby accessories are always adorned with crystals. Baby shoes for infants are completely blinged out—including the soles. Once a child begins to walk, only the tops of the shoes are crystallized. *Courtesy of Mark Johnson*

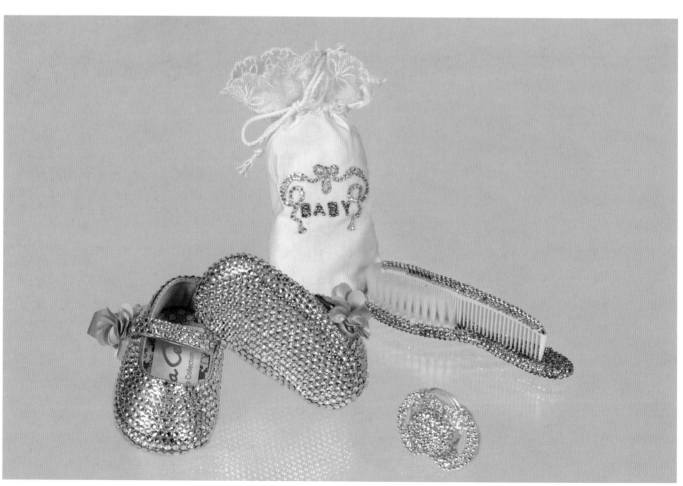

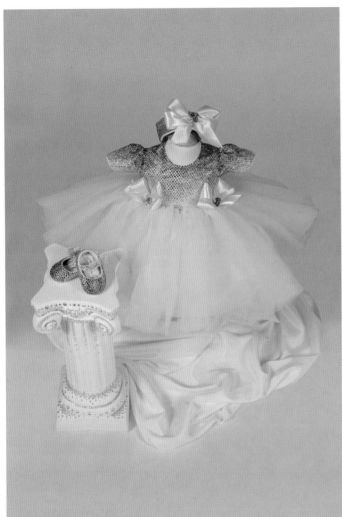
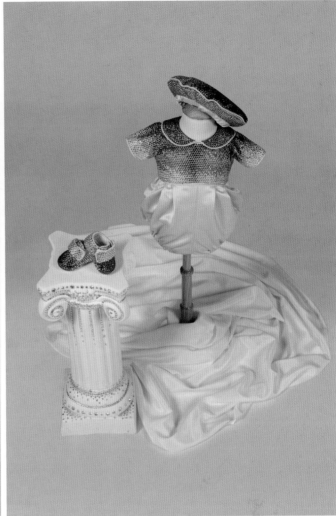

There are many celebrations throughout the year for which Gypsies and Travelers will order special outfits from me. But no matter what the event, it's go big and go bling or go home. Why do they order such over-the-top designs? For the same reason you might buy a designer handbag or boast about the college your child attends. It's about getting attention, promoting one's status, and in the community, it can also mean potential matchmaking. There's an unspoken (but highly intense) competition that exists to prove to others how well off a family is, how great the head of household is as a provider, and what a terrific catch a son or daughter could be. Generally, women are brought up to marry, keep a clean home, and raise the kids while the men work and bring home the money. When a special occasion arises, they order opulent outfits to visually signal their family's wealth and success to others.

For example, when a child is born, the parents go all out. A typical custom layette for a newborn usually includes matching crib bumpers and skirt, a baby blanket plus matching mommy and baby robes, a baby bottle wrap, a pacifier, and other accessories. The infant's monogram or some themed decoration is also ordered to hang on the hospital room door proudly announcing the new arrival. In addition, a few coordinating baby ensembles are made up and put on display around the hospital room to show off the newborn's bling couture. Of course, Dad and any siblings also order coordinating bling tops to wear during hospital visits.

Newborn baby "bubbles." "Hers" comes with matching headband; "His" comes with matching tam. Each includes coordinating shoes. *Courtesy of Mark Johnson*

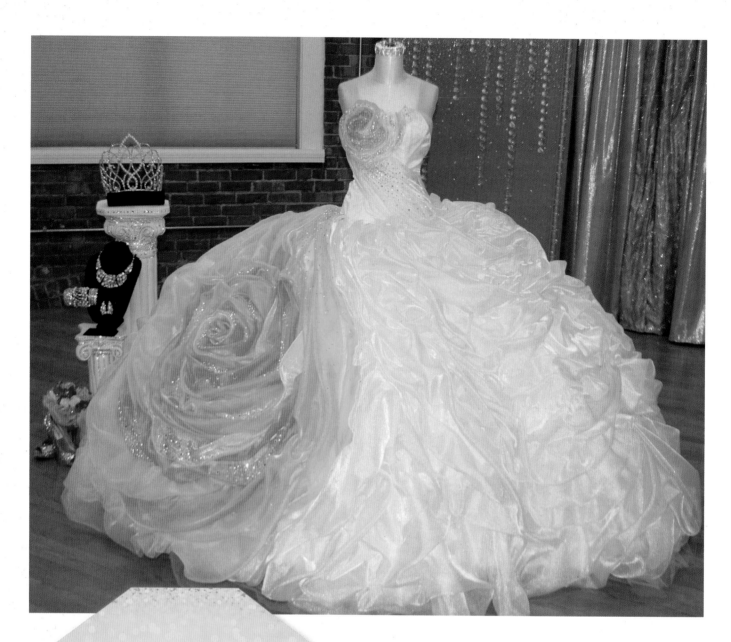

Courtesy of Tisi Farrar

Opposite Gypsy wedding gowns almost always feature a sweetheart neckline corset that laces up the back. This color would be known as "Windex blue" on the Gypsy color preference chart. *Courtesy of Tisi Farrar*

Crystal Clear

On the average, my Gypsy-style dresses usually weigh about 80 pounds. For this "orange sherbet swirl" creation, I combined 100 yards of ivory, tangerine, and peach organza. Two specially crafted petticoats give the skirt volume. My "delicious" creation boasts 12,000 Swarovski® stones in Sun, Peach, and Aurora Borealis, plus Swarovski® pearl accents.

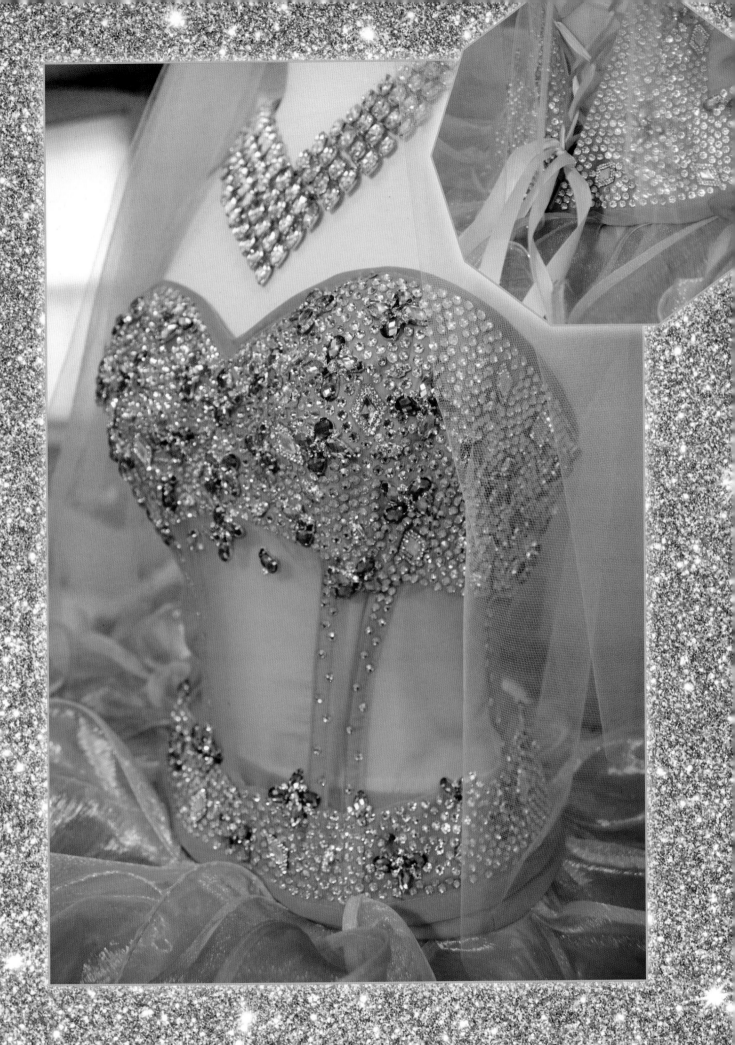

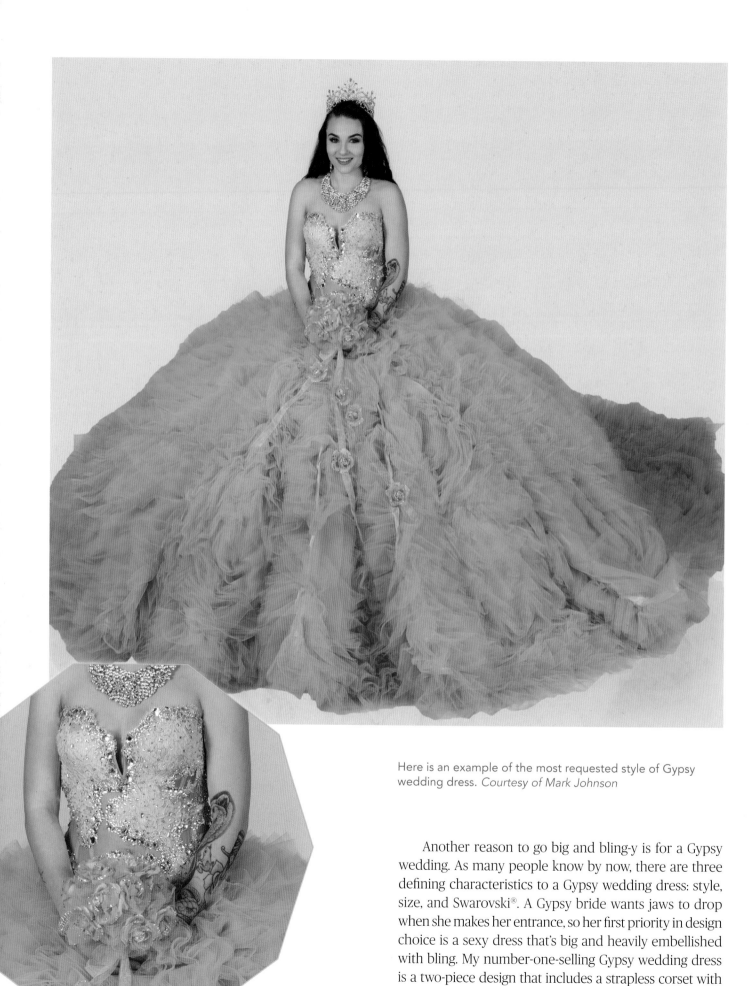

Here is an example of the most requested style of Gypsy wedding dress. *Courtesy of Mark Johnson*

Another reason to go big and bling-y is for a Gypsy wedding. As many people know by now, there are three defining characteristics to a Gypsy wedding dress: style, size, and Swarovski®. A Gypsy bride wants jaws to drop when she makes her entrance, so her first priority in design choice is a sexy dress that's big and heavily embellished with bling. My number-one-selling Gypsy wedding dress is a two-piece design that includes a strapless corset with

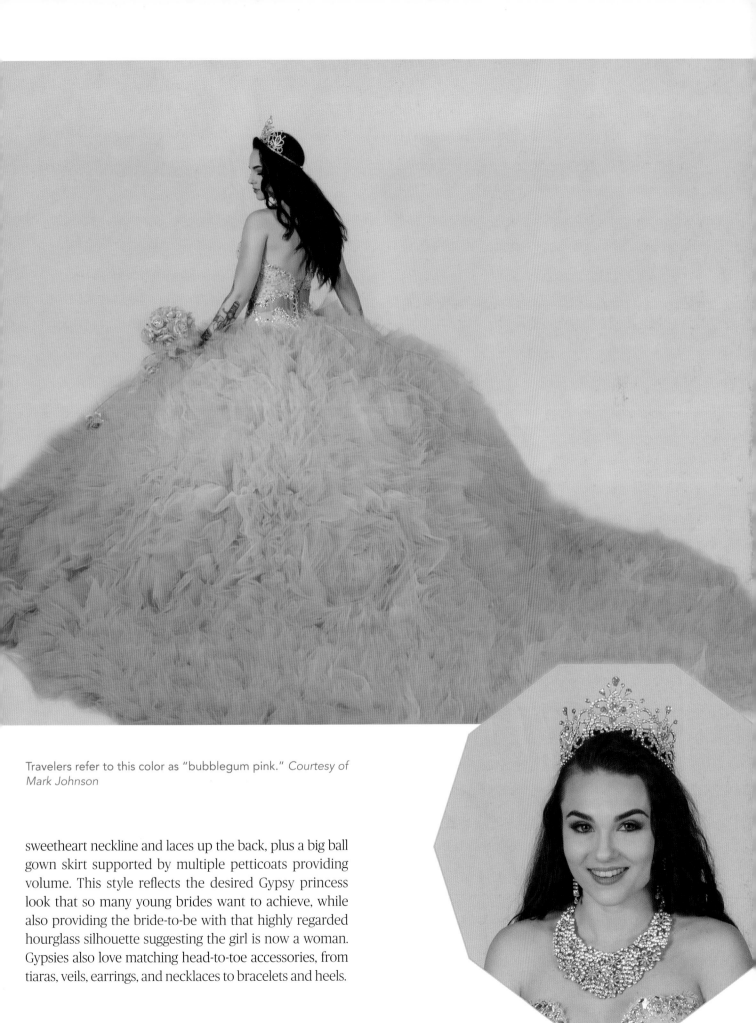

Travelers refer to this color as "bubblegum pink." *Courtesy of Mark Johnson*

sweetheart neckline and laces up the back, plus a big ball gown skirt supported by multiple petticoats providing volume. This style reflects the desired Gypsy princess look that so many young brides want to achieve, while also providing the bride-to-be with that highly regarded hourglass silhouette suggesting the girl is now a woman. Gypsies also love matching head-to-toe accessories, from tiaras, veils, earrings, and necklaces to bracelets and heels.

Other events that my Traveler clients order custom crystal couture for include baptisms, birthdays, first communions, funerals, Easter, Halloween, Christmas, and car parties. Yes, I said car parties. My Traveler clients like to celebrate whenever they purchase a new car, and they do that by throwing it (the car) a party. The car is parked outside the home, and the entire community is invited to stop by to view it while the proud owner and family pose, all decked out in coordinating car-themed blingwear.

No matter what my Traveler clients order, I can guarantee the finished work will incorporate bright colors. I have learned that they have their own unique color preferences, incorporating hot hues with descriptive titles such as bubblegum pink, Windex blue, taxi yellow, Palmolive green, and fire engine red. When I get a call and am asked to design a "taxi" yellow dress, I know that means they want fabric that is brighter than a lemon but not as light as canary yellow.

I love working with both my Traveler and Gypsy clients because they give me creative freedom. They love vibrant colors, unique materials, and daring designs. They are "design courageous," always game to do what's never been done before. It's so much fun to be able to color outside the lines when we collaborate on designs.

In some cases I am dressing my third generation of Traveler and Gypsy families. I think my successful partnership with those communities is partly because I understand their fashion priorities. I offer them what they want–daring creativity, vibrant colors, and lots of bling. More importantly, we have a mutual respect for one another. They appreciate my honesty, confidentiality, directness, and reliability. And they appreciate my team's ability to turn around last-minute orders if need be.

I feel very fortunate to have close relationships with many Gypsy and Traveler families. I have been invited into their homes and have attended many of their family celebrations. Today I have over 4,400 contacts in my phone. Most of them are more than just clients: they are friends.

One thing I greatly admire about my clients is that they are extremely family oriented and loyal to one another. Children are the center of attention and main focus of their parents' lives. They want only the very best for their kids and will often sacrifice to give them just that. Extended family members are also part of the tight bond and share a strong pride in the family's heritage.

Crystal Clear

I had a major design dilemma a few years ago when a Traveler client called me to design eighty-seven tops for several families throwing a combined car party. Sixteen cars were being featured at one showing. A cardinal rule in their society is that no one gets caught wearing the same design. Thus, every one of the eighty-seven tops had to be a unique style while incorporating only the three colors of the cars being feted: red, black, and silver. I spent days slashing, fringing, blinging, embellishing, layering, and cutting tops. I used every design technique I ever learned, and the eighty-seven finished tops were big hits at the party.

There is some competition out there for creating bling designs for the Gypsy and Traveler communities. A handful of individuals have actually tried to knock off my designs, but the difference in quality (and price point) is obvious. You won't find sloppy hems, unfinished trims, or mismatched colors on an authentic Sondra Celli. My staff consists of expert designers and veteran seamstresses, and therefore we turn out extraordinary one-of-a-kind pieces that are more complicated to create. (A number of clients have even referred to my designs as "architectural wonders"!) The competition usually puts out standard and uninspired cookie-cutter dresses because they are simpler, quicker, and cheaper to make. We never cut corners with inexpensive fabrics, fake feathers, or plastic stones.

Yet another thing that sets us apart is that we can turn out orders on very short notice. Among the many clients I work with, it is not unusual for a huge party to pop up at the last minute and for rush orders to pour into my office.

Although I have been designing for the Gypsy and Traveler communities for over thirty-five years, I have been creating designs on TLC's *My Big Fat American Gypsy Wedding* for only six years. In that short time, I have seen Gypsy-style fashions go mainstream. I get calls from non-Gypsies who live all over the world wanting to order dresses they've seen on the show–and not just for weddings. They want Gypsy-style dresses for proms, quinceañeras, and even baptisms and communions. They love the dramatic designs and bling. The popularity

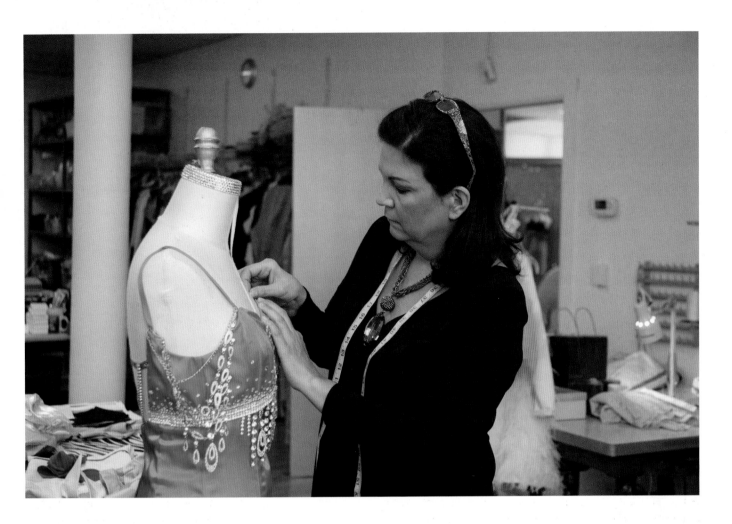

of my dresses has spread the world over, and I was approached by an entrepreneurial businessman from the United Kingdom who wanted to have one of my designs transformed into a limited-edition figurine called *Crystal Bride*. It is rendered by hand by a renowned master sculptor with the Royal Staffordshire Company. The bride shimmers with a hand-painted platinum tiara, thirty-one handmade flowers, and sparkling Swarovski® crystal accents. Truly exquisite.

Above Courtesy of Sondra Celli

Below Limited-edition *Crystal Bride by Sondra Celli* is handcrafted in English fine bone china. Each figurine comes signed and numbered and includes a certificate of authenticity. *Courtesy of Tisi Farrar*

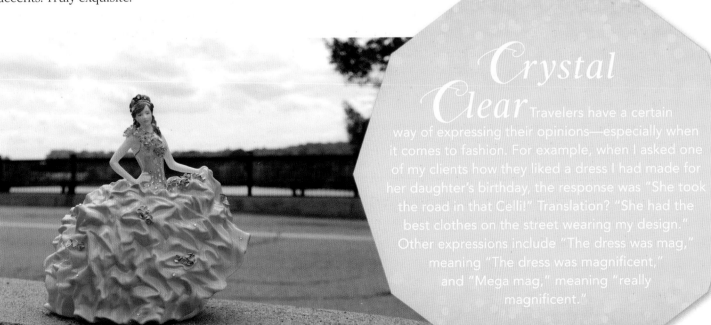

Crystal Clear

Travelers have a certain way of expressing their opinions—especially when it comes to fashion. For example, when I asked one of my clients how they liked a dress I had made for her daughter's birthday, the response was "She took the road in that Celli!" Translation? "She had the best clothes on the street wearing my design." Other expressions include "The dress was mag," meaning "The dress was magnificent," and "Mega mag," meaning "really magnificent."

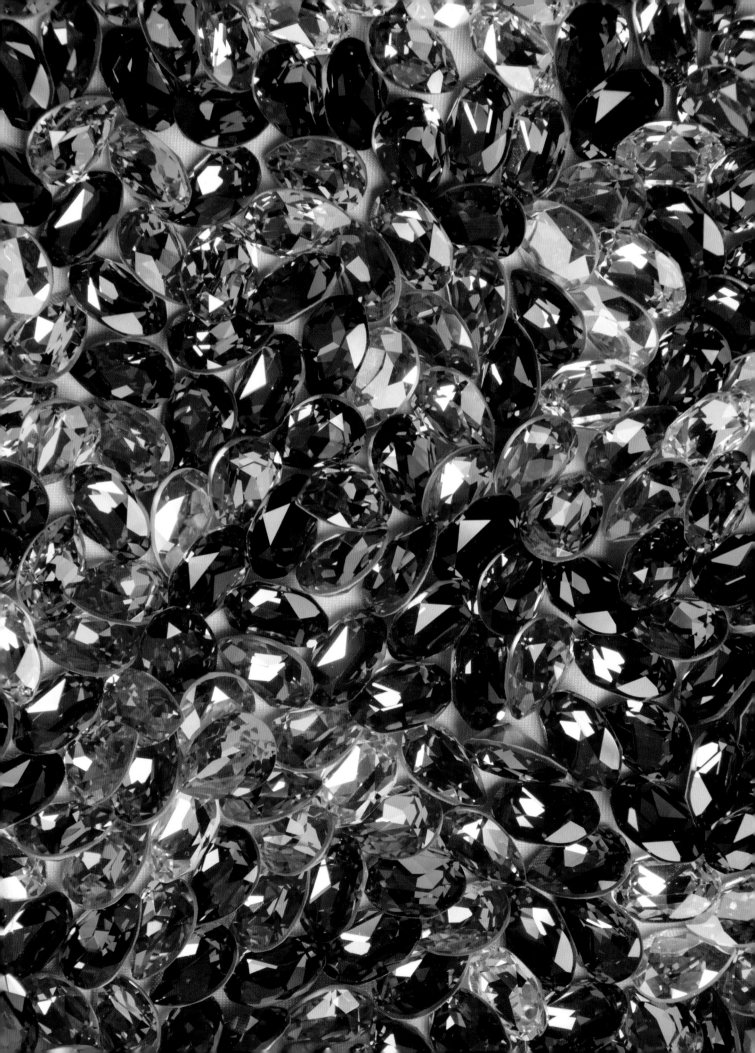

5.
Behind the Scenes

Over the years I have designed dresses using real flowers, real candy, and real dollars, and I've even wired up a pair of wings and several gowns so they would light up. Every episode of *My Big Fat American Gypsy Wedding* is a unique (and sometimes daunting) design challenge, but I love having my design skills tested and being able to make bold decisions.

When producers were searching for a designer to star in the US version of the popular UK series *My Big Fat Gypsy Wedding*, word of mouth led them to me. The producers had called around the Gypsy communities and my name kept popping up. Although I design for everyone, I have had a very large number of Romanichal and Irish Traveler clients for decades. I was thrilled when the network asked me to be the designer for *My Big Fat American Gypsy Wedding*. I just didn't know what I was getting into.

The TV show's production company, which is based in London, books all the Gypsy brides featured on the show. Once a bride-to-be is confirmed for the show, the

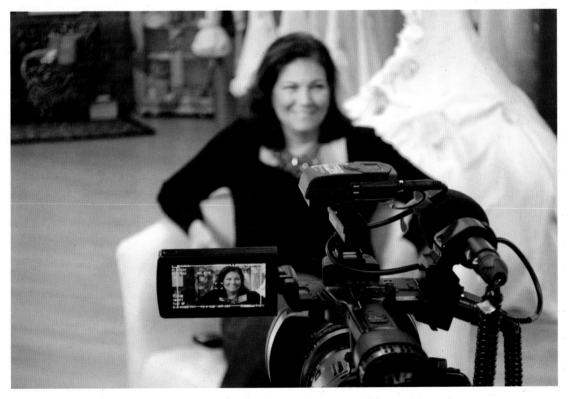

Courtesy of Mark Johnson

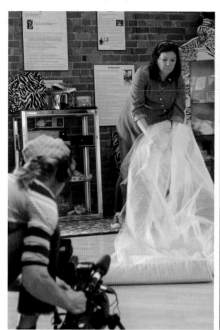
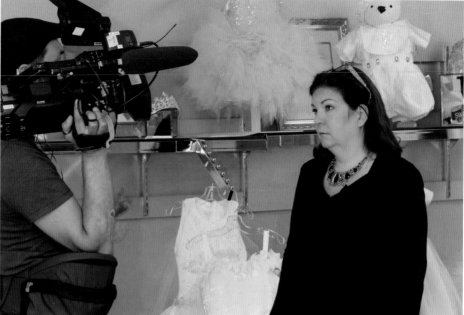

producers send me a name and maybe a sentence or two about how the couple met. Next, a phone call is set up between me and the bride-to-be so we can discuss design ideas and get her measurements. The phone call, however, is usually scheduled just days away from the wedding. This can be a bit stressful for me, since it allows no time for mistakes. There are even times where I have had to produce a gigantic Gypsy gown almost overnight, which, I probably don't have to tell you, is a remarkable feat.

What also adds to the stress level is the fact that I don't close up my shop to shoot these episodes. It is a matter of running my business as usual while I am simultaneously shooting a reality TV show. That means that every Gypsy dress design featured on *My Big Fat American Gypsy Wedding* has to be worked into and around already scheduled orders. This is where multitasking comes in handy.

A typical shoot day has me arriving at six o'clock in the morning for hair and makeup, then organizing my staff so that they know what designs they'll be working on. Next, the production crew arrives and sets up while I catch up on paperwork until taping begins. In between takes, I'll answer texts, emails, and questions from my staff; rework my schedule; accept deliveries; and do whatever quick tasks I can fit in. The shoot day typically ends around six o'clock at night.

Crystal Clear The benefit of using tulle to make a bridal gown is that it is lightweight and cost effective, and enough of it will give you that princess look that most young brides are looking for. My Gypsy-style dresses usually feature skirts made with an average of 500 yards of tulle. That is about five times the length of a football field!

Left Crew shoots footage for the show. *Courtesy of Mark Johnson*

Right Discussing production details before shooting. *Courtesy of Mark Johnson*

Opposite Seventeen colors of tulle were cut into thousands of small strips to create this rainbow mermaid gown. The colorful pieces were sewn together by six seamstresses over a two-day period to make the dress skirt and train. *Courtesy of Mark Johnson*

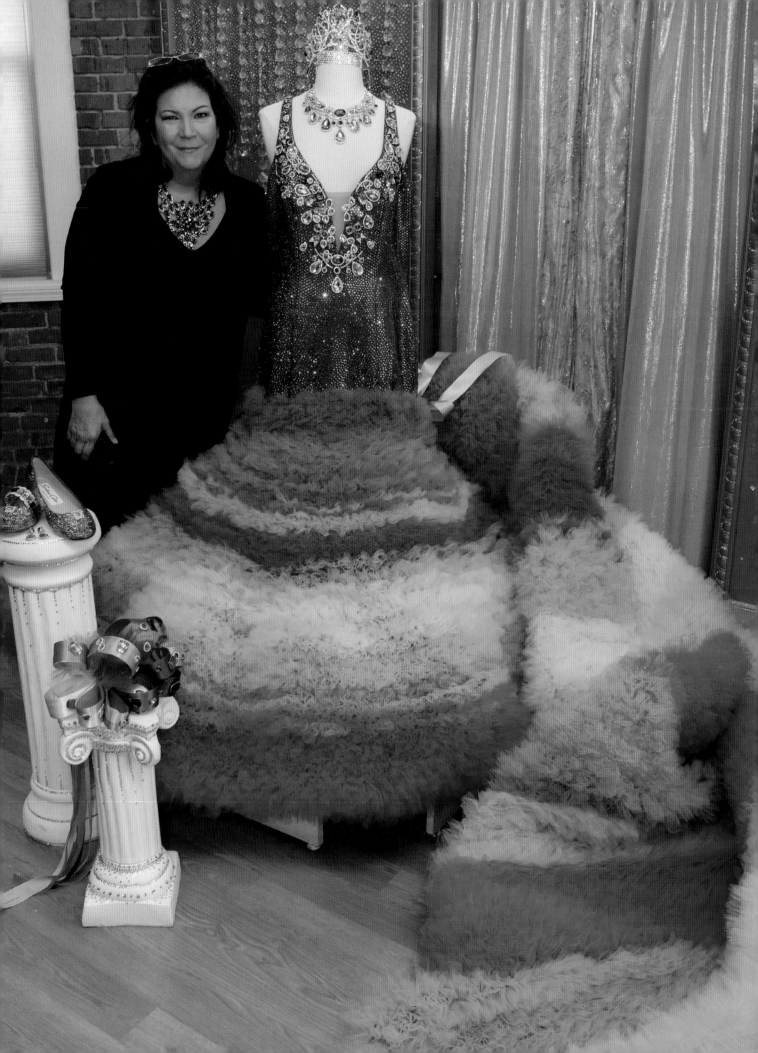

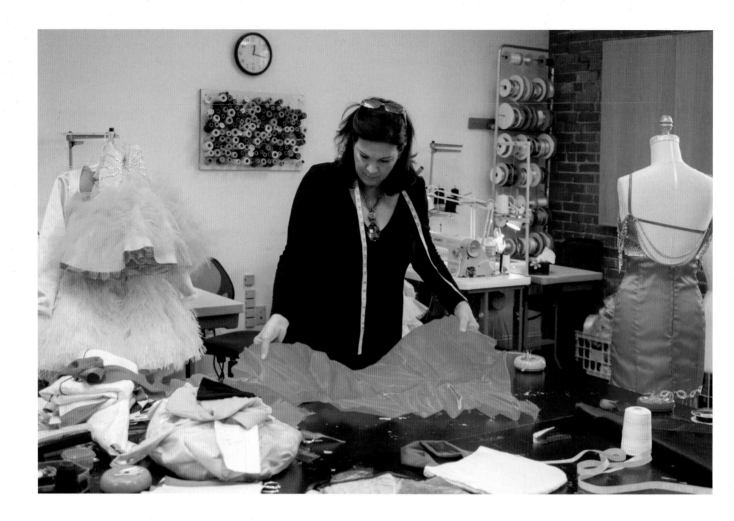

The dress designs for *My Big Fat American Gypsy Wedding* are a combination of what the Gypsy bride-to-be originally wants and my interpretation of that vision. Once a style of gown is agreed on, I order in all the fabrics, notions, and embellishments–usually via overnight delivery, since I rarely get advance notice of these custom Gypsy-style dress orders. Once the materials arrive, Mira, my brilliant designer/seamstress who has worked with me for years, begins to assemble the dress. Part of that job entails creating multiple custom petticoats to be worn underneath to provide support and volume.

Special touches such as handmade flowers might be added to the design. Mira and Carol (another amazingly talented staff member) usually work on those items as well as on any matching accessories such as bouquets, masks, tiaras, headpieces, jewelry, and shoes.

The final embellishments are done by the "Bling-ettes." That's how we lovingly refer to my staff of highly skilled artistic designers who do the crystal work. Their job is painstaking and precise and can take anywhere from several hours to several months to complete.

If the dress we are making for the show is an especially time-consuming design, I will assign three or more Bling-ettes to that one dress to get it done. The dress is spread out on a work table, and each girl takes an area and starts adding the stones. Every stone is placed by hand, one by one.

A basic Gypsy bridal ensemble featured on *My Big Fat American Gypsy Wedding* usually includes a bodice with sweetheart neckline and large skirt over multiple petticoats. Accessories include a tiara, veil, matching jewelry, shoes, and bouquet. The average cost of a dress featured on the show starts at $10,000 and goes up based on design, materials used, and amount of bling.

Above I oversee all the pattern work and do most of the pattern cutting for every design we make. *Courtesy of Mark Johnson*

Opposite top Mira expertly embellishes a corset with assorted jewelry pieces. *Courtesy of Tisi Farrar*

Opposite bottom Mira often gets lost in tulle while creating our custom petticoats. *Courtesy of Tisi Farrar*

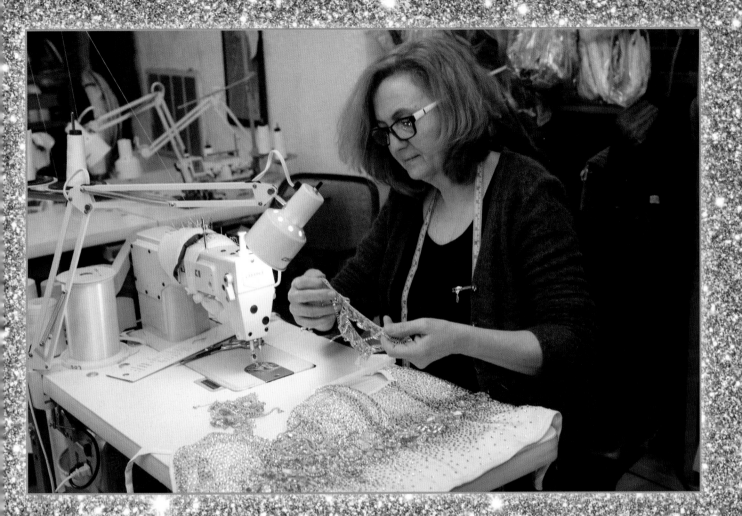

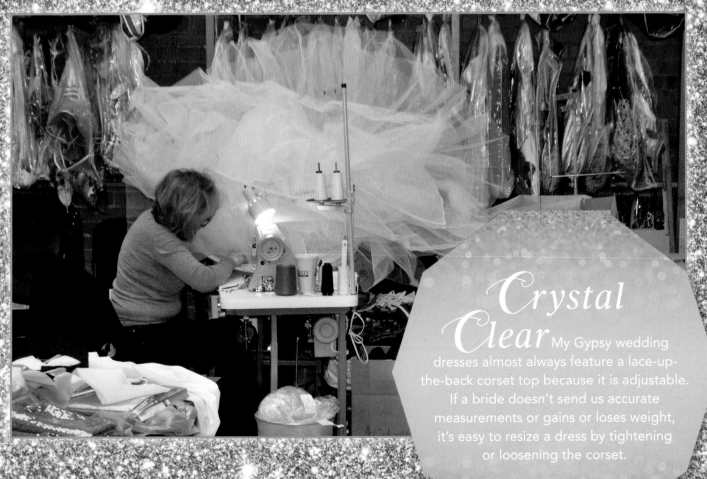

Crystal Clear

My Gypsy wedding dresses almost always feature a lace-up-the-back corset top because it is adjustable. If a bride doesn't send us accurate measurements or gains or loses weight, it's easy to resize a dress by tightening or loosening the corset.

Whenever we finish a design for the show, we put the dress on a mannequin in our showroom and display the matching accessories around it for "the big reveal." That's when we bring the bride into my shop to view her dress for the very first time.

When the bride arrives, she is met at the door and immediately blindfolded, along with anyone traveling with her. I lead everyone into the showroom and position them directly in front of the display. Once cameras start rolling, I order everyone to remove their blindfolds, and the crew captures everyone's reactions. The brides are usually nervous before the big reveal and, to tell the truth, so am I. The last thing I want is for a bride to be unhappy about her wedding dress–especially when her reaction is going to be televised. So far, thank goodness, I have an exemplary track record of pleasing the brides.

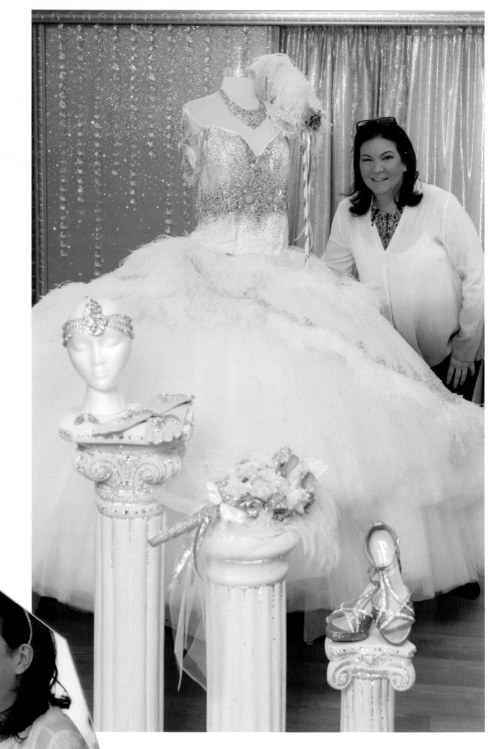

Above This white-and-gold Gypsy-style wedding ensemble featured on the show consists of a necklace, corset, tulle skirt, and handheld masquerade mask with ostrich plume. Displayed in front on columns (*left to right*) are matching accessories: headband, earrings, gloves, bouquet, and heels. *Courtesy of Mark Johnson*

Left A nervous Gypsy bride waits for the signal to remove her blindfold. She will be seeing her wedding dress for the very first time. *Courtesy of Mark Johnson*

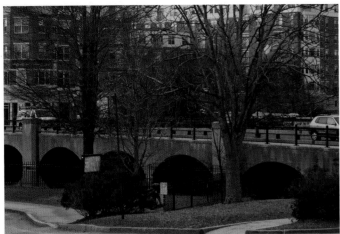

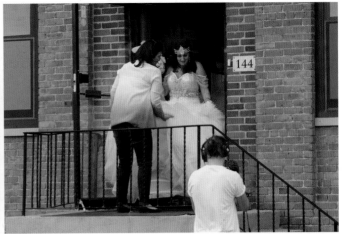

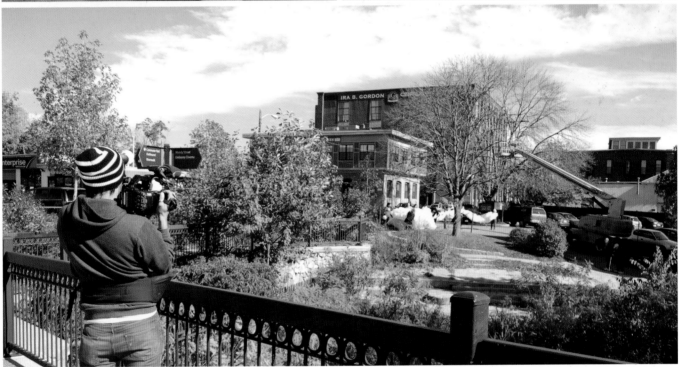

After the reveal is out of the way, the bride tries on her dress and all her accessories. Once she's wearing her Gypsy finery, we then head out to "Gypsy Bridge" for a walk around the neighborhood to test out the fit and maneuverability. (It's not the official name of the bridge. We call it that because of the number of Gypsy brides who we have had walk across it.) The test walk (or "walkabout") allows the brides to get used to the feel, size, and weight of the gown. It can be especially difficult while balancing on five-inch heels and trying to keep a six-inch crown steady on the head. Volunteers from my staff or family members of the bride (or both) walk along to help support the dress train.

If you are in the area and time it right, you might catch a jaw-dropping Gypsy Wedding fashion show parading down the street.

The routine is to head out of the shop, cross over Gypsy Bridge, walk through a bit of the downtown area past a few shops, cross the street and walk down the other side of the bridge, and then repeat the "walkabout." We usually complete two or three loops before heading back.

Top left "Gypsy Bridge" is located directly outside my front door. *Courtesy of Mark Johnson*

Top right Sometimes just getting out the door in a Gypsy wedding gown can be a chore. *Courtesy of Tisi Farrar*

Bottom Videographer on Gypsy Bridge shoots a bride leaving my shop for her test walk. *Courtesy of Tisi Farrar*

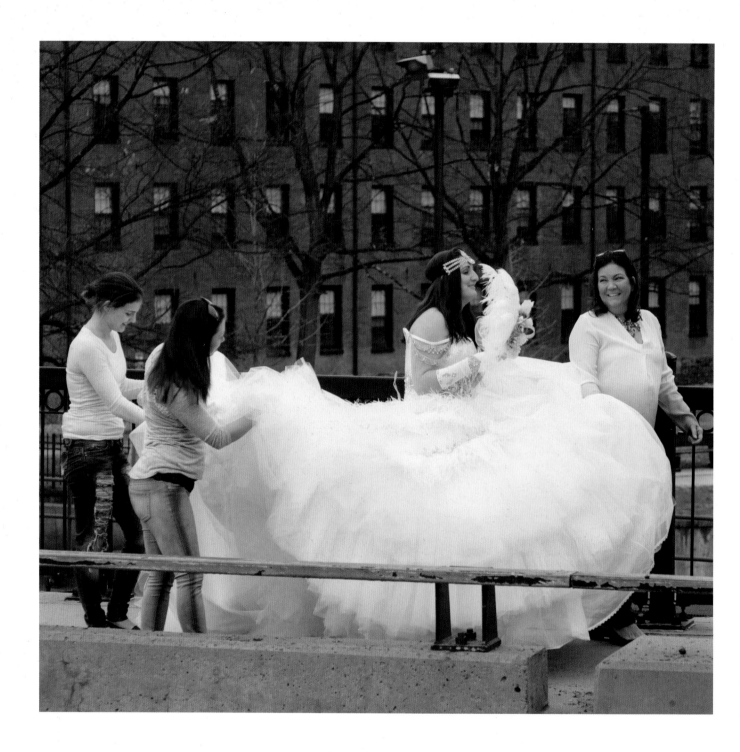

The best part of the walkabout is catching reactions from passersby, motorists, and store vendors as the big, blinged-out ball gown goes by. The sparkling spectacle elicits whistles, hoots, honking horns, comical double-takes, applause, and lots of enthusiastic thumbs ups. Check out these photos from a few of our Gypsy Bridge expeditions . . .

Above Crossing Gypsy Bridge. *Courtesy of Tisi Farrar*

Opposite top Courtesy of Tisi Farrar

Opposite bottom A fan stops us for a quick photo. *Courtesy of Sondra Celli*

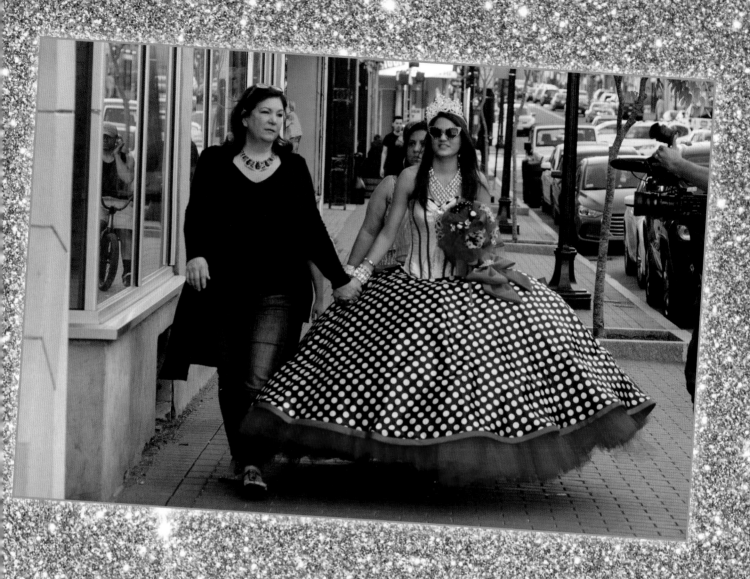
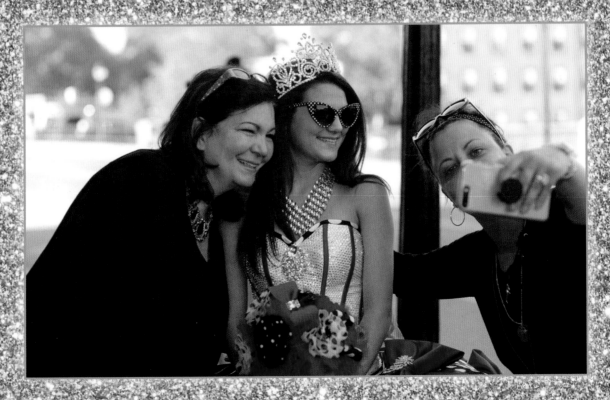

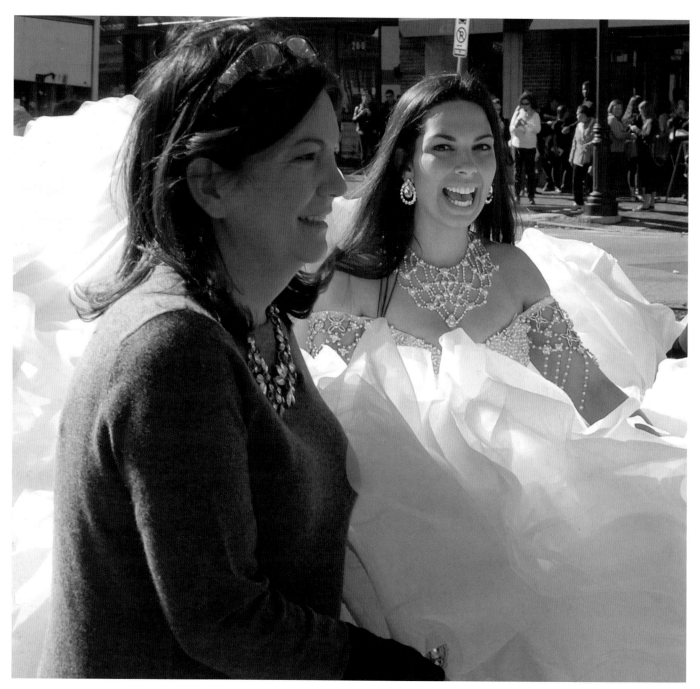

Courtesy of Sondra Celli

After returning to the shop, if there are no alterations to be made to the gown, the bride-to-be changes back into her street clothes and heads home. Meanwhile, we pack everything up and have it shipped to the producers, who will be shooting the actual wedding and reception.

Packing up one of my Gypsy-style wedding dresses for shipping can be a bit of a physical ordeal. It usually takes two people to handle the packing of the refrigerator-sized boxes. The tulle or hoop petticoats are stuffed into one box while the corset, skirt, and all the accessories are packed into another box. The skirt is inverted so that the waist goes in first. Someone then folds the skirt into thirds and hugs it together (making it less voluminous) while the other person guides it into the box. (Sounds complicated, but we now have it down to a science.) We label the boxes, weigh them, and ship them off.

Quite often I am asked to attend the weddings of my Gypsy brides, and if my production schedule allows, I will

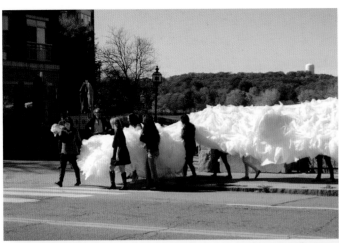
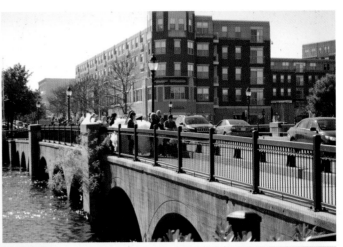
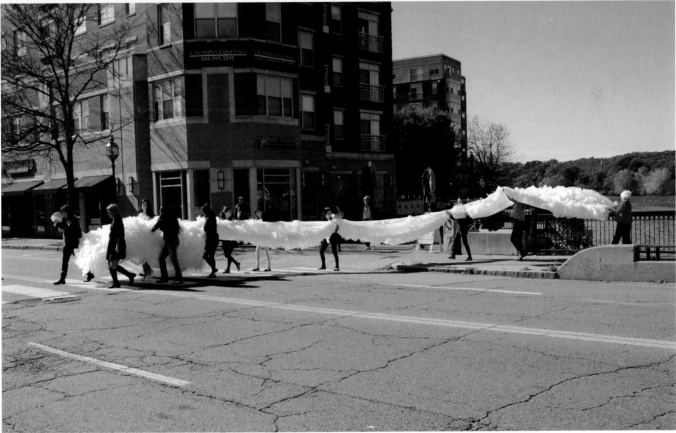

attend the wedding. Whenever I do go, I always pack my little black bag just in case of any wardrobe malfunctions. The bag contains threads, needles, scissors, pins, and other emergency tools of the trade.

What happens to these blinding bling-packed dresses after the wedding? Usually Gypsies sell them to other Gypsies or pull all the stones off and use them to embellish other things, but once in a great while, you might find one of my designs for sale online.

Why did the Gypsy bride cross the road? To get to the other side, of course! This was the biggest and most expensive dress I ever made. You will find more shots of this gigantic dress later in the book. *Courtesy of Tisi Farrar*

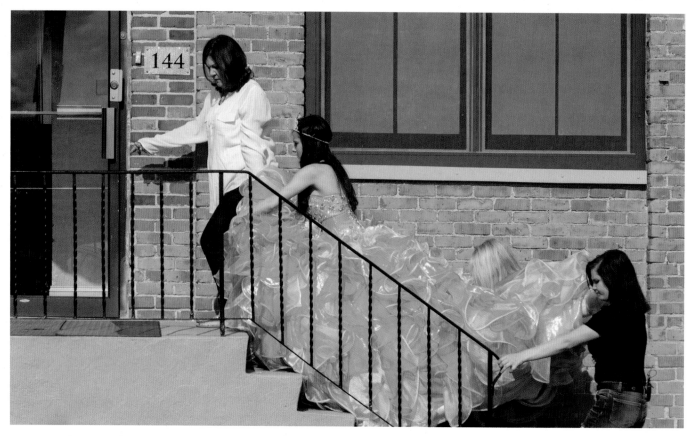

Courtesy of Tisi Farrar

Sometimes we encounter unexpected bumps in the road during the filming of *My Big Fat American Gypsy Wedding*. I have encountered my fair share of them and have had to think fast and act quickly because the show must always go on.

A Few Behind-the-Scenes Blooper Moments...

I had scheduled one of the Bling-ettes to completely pack a white, strapless bustier with thousands of crystals. It was to ship out the next day. Packing a design is a time-consuming process because each of the stones is applied by hand, one by one, and placed tightly together. In an unguarded moment, she accidentally knocked over her energy drink, drenching the white bustier with her bright-red drink. It seemed as if time stood still. I quickly grabbed the saturated bustier and tried washing it, then bleaching

it, but the stain would not come out. A new bustier had to be created, and I put the entire team to work on it and on packing it with stones until 2 a.m. The damaged bustier was a total loss. I tossed it out, watching about $2,000 go down the drain. Today, all beverages (except water) are now banished from the workroom.

One of my Gypsy brides wanted "Biker Chic" for her bridal outfit because she was going to ride off into the sunset on a motorcycle with her new husband. I created a custom pair of sexy, skinny-legged pants in stretchy silver lamé with zipper accents at the ankles and paired them with a matching lamé bodice packed with Clear crystals and topped with a biker jacket. A sparkling crystal belt at the waist featured a detachable pink tulle skirt lined in pink satin. When the display was

Which look would you have chosen for a "biker chic" wedding?

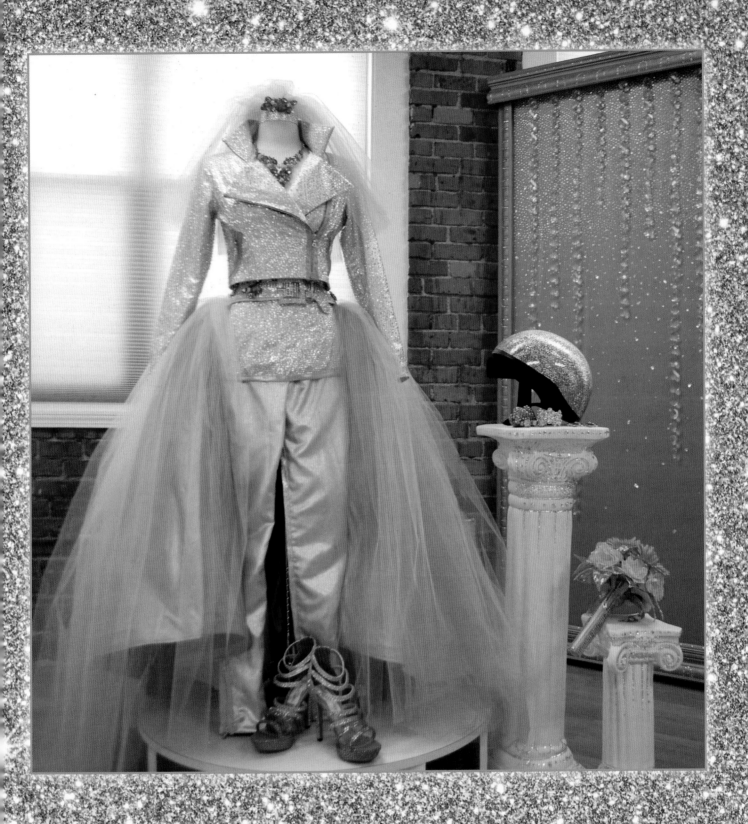

Sexy pants...

…or tulle skirt?

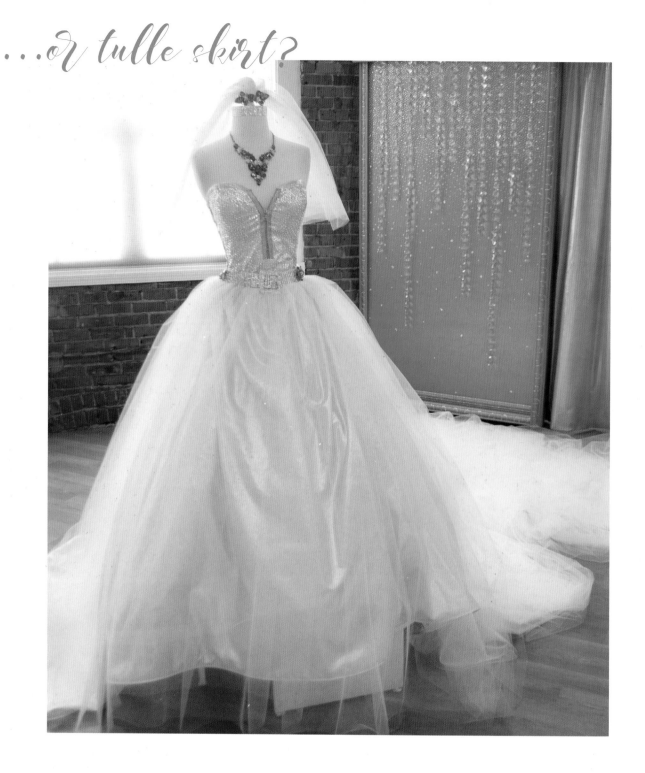

revealed to the bride and her mother-in-law, the bride squealed with delight at my creation, but the mother-in-law applied the breaks. She was not at all impressed and demanded a more traditional look. I had to ditch the pants and quickly created a silver lamé skirt with tulle overlay and a twenty-foot train accented with crystals. After all that, the motorcycle ride into the sunset never happened.

 I received a call from a customer who wanted me to make a cupcake dress for her six-year-old daughter to wear to a Halloween party. The design needed to be made of lightweight materials so that the skirt of the dress would not cave in or weigh her down. The hardware store held the answer! I made dozens of cupcakes by using spray insulation foam, and then used spackle as frosting, which I colored with food dye. Crystals were then added as "sprinkles" to decorate the faux cupcakes. In addition, I custom designed a special petticoat by using horsehair, which is a sturdy yet flexible netting that provides support and volume. It worked perfectly and the dress was a sweet success!

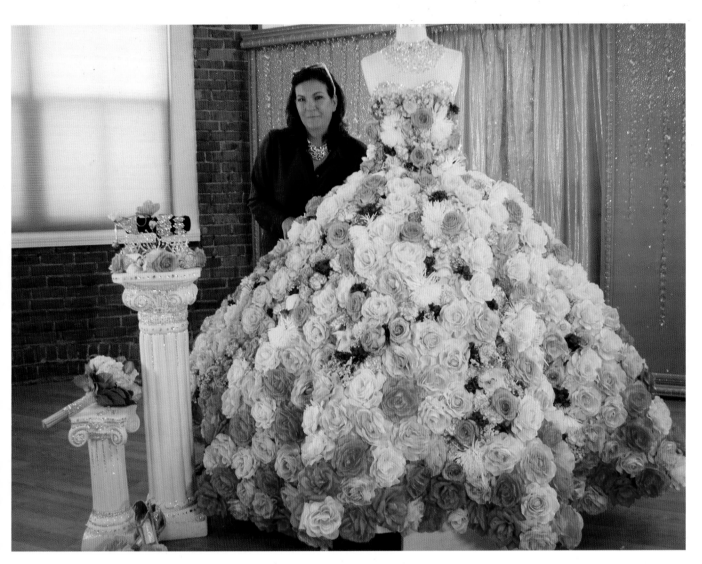

This is what I call real "Flower Power"! *Courtesy of Tisi Farrar*

If you are a fan of *My Big Fat American Gypsy Wedding*, then you know we sometimes run into a few problems when trying to create a Gypsy bride's dream dress. One bride-to-be ordered a dress made with real flowers. This would be a first for her and for me. She wanted *Gerbera* daisies to be used, but they were bulky and too difficult to handle. We settled on roses, dahlias, *Cymbidium* orchids, popcorn hydrangeas, carnations, and dianthus. Double-sided floral tape adheres the blossoms to the Duchess satin dress. The finished design was extraordinary, but keeping the flowers fresh for the wedding was key. Our plan was to transport the dress in a van with the air conditioner on full blast during the fourteen-hour road trip. Unfortunately, the van's air conditioner blew up partway through the trip, and the dress did not fare well. Upon arrival, many of the blossoms had wilted, while others had turned brown. Now what? I received a call from the frantic bride-to-be and assured her that I would take care of her fashion emergency. I immediately booked a flight for myself and expert designer and seamstress Mira to fly down to repair the dress. I then called ahead and had a production assistant run out to local florists and supermarkets to purchase fresh replacement flowers.

When Mira and I arrived in our hotel room, fresh flowers were waiting. We immediately went to work replacing the dead flowers until the wee hours of the morning. It could have been one big floral failure, but we managed to rework the dress in time for the wedding and ended up smelling like roses.

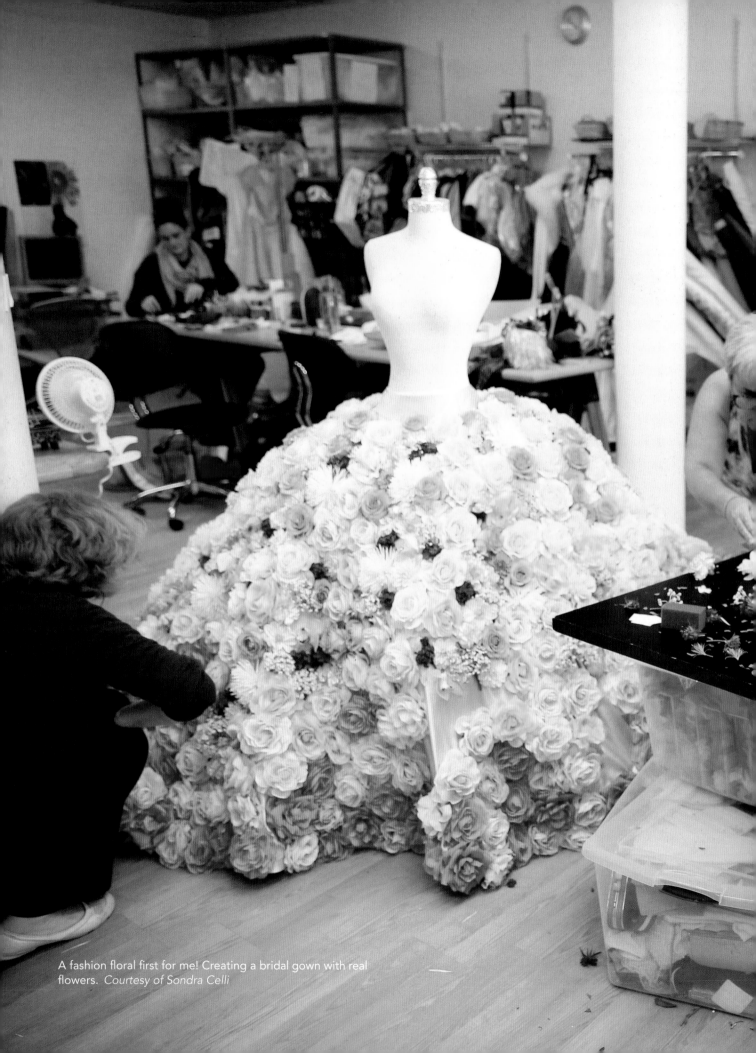

A fashion floral first for me! Creating a bridal gown with real flowers. *Courtesy of Sondra Celli*

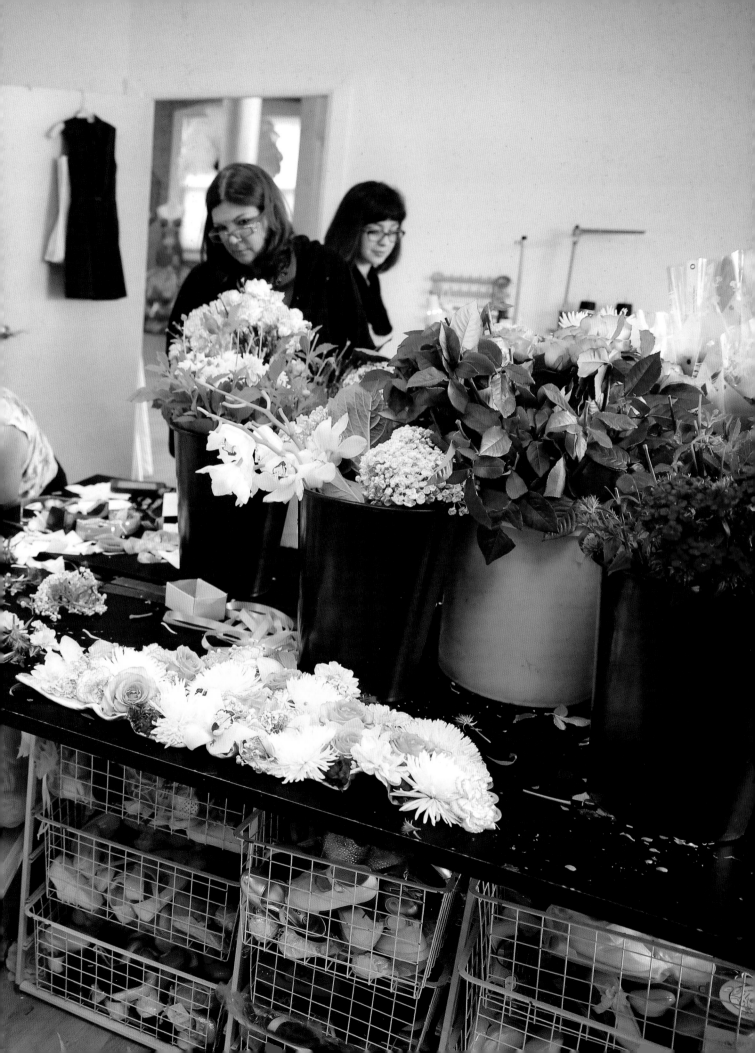

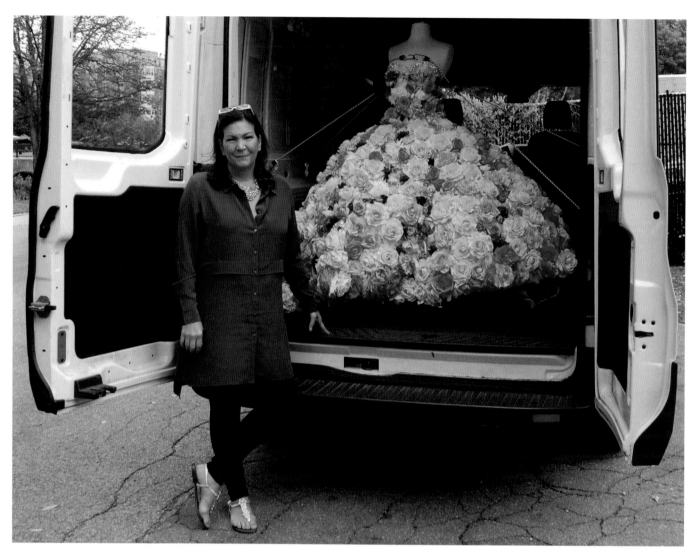

The dress was loaded and securely strapped into a van for transport with the air conditioner blasting! *Courtesy of Tisi Farrar*

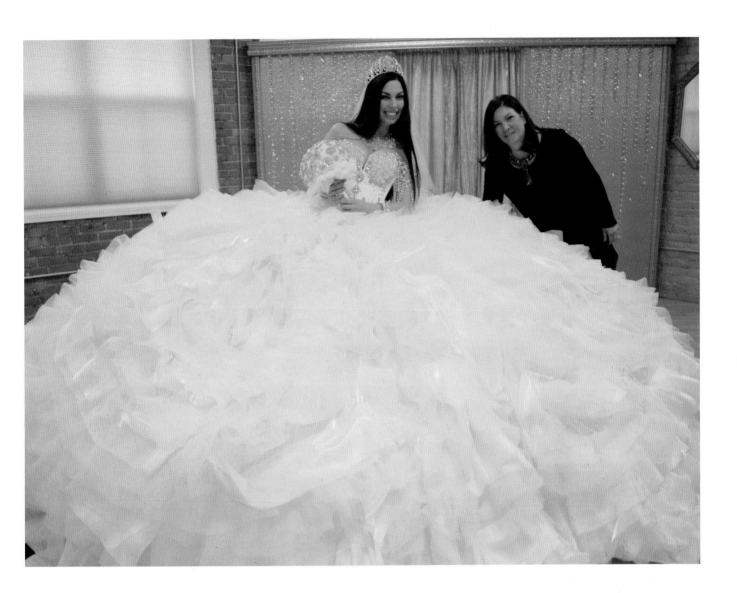

Bigger Than Big

The biggest dress ever commissioned in my career to date was for Tatiana, a Gypsy of Greek heritage. She wanted the biggest and most memorable dress ever. She got it. We designed eight custom petticoats, using 500 feet of special industrial tubing to support the ginormous dress. Six hundred yards of sparkle satin and over 400 yards of white silk organza made up the dress and 150-yard-long train. The dress was embellished with over 50,000 crystals and would end up weighing 100 pounds. We had to use six refrigerator-sized boxes to ship the dress and accessories. A special flatbed truck was hired to transport the bride to the church. To get a perfect perspective on the size of the design, the show's producers used a camera drone to get a sky-eye view! At a cost of $40,000, it was the most expensive dress I have ever created.

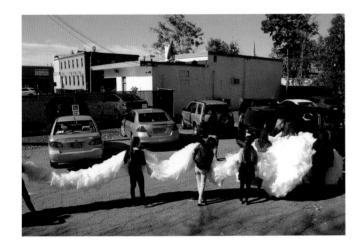

Top Beautiful Gypsy bride Tatiana asked for "the biggest dress ever" and she got it! *Courtesy of Tisi Farrar*

Above Attempting to get the bride and her dress into a car was a bust. In the end, Tatiana had to be driven to her ceremony in the back of a flatbed truck. *Courtesy of Tisi Farrar*

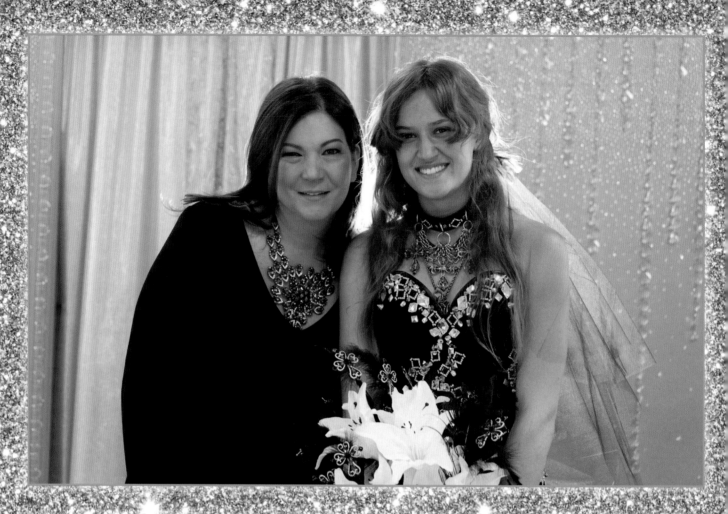
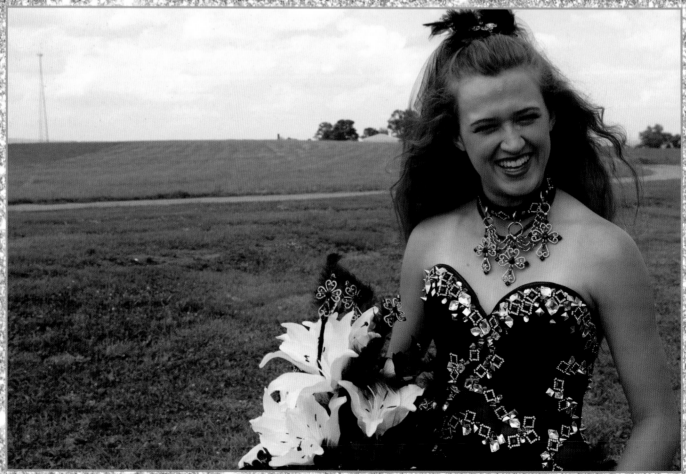

Here Comes the Bride, All Dressed in . . . Black?

I had a Gypsy bride client who was a tomboy with a taste for "goth"–a style usually characterized by black clothing, metal, and leather accessories. The mother of the bride wanted a traditional, poufy, princess-style dress for her daughter. I prevented a wardrobe war by making a glamorous gothic-style gown that they both loved! It was a black lace corset with sheer mesh, leather trim accented with Swarovski® crystal chunky stones, metal silver spikes, and studs. A specially designed crinoline petticoat gave shape to the high/low skirt, made from tattered tulle and 1,100 turkey feathers individually applied. Her accessories included heavy black boots with silver spikes, nailheads, and gothic crosses; a black, open-weave hose; a leather dog collar with spikes and gothic crosses; a chunky crystal bracelet and spiked leather cuffs; a short, torn, black tulle veil with turkey feathers; and a gothic cross brooch secured to a hair comb. She carried a bouquet of white calla lilies, black lilies of the valley hand-painted with fabric dye, more gothic crosses, and turkey feathers all wrapped with a black silk ribbon and accented with spikes on the handle.

Fashion Freeze

One brutal Boston winter, we were designing a winter wonderland gown for a Gypsy bride to be featured on *My Big Fat American Gypsy Wedding*. It was an over-the-top design, for which we are known, but the added problem was that we had lost heat at the shop. It was freezing inside, but the dress had to be finished for filming the next day. My entire staff worked late into the night dressed in coats, hats, and fingerless gloves while several space heaters cranked heat. The girls suffered through blinging out a hooded jacket packed with 8,000 Clear Swarovski® crystals meant to look like ice. A huge muff was packed with 20,000 stones. The dress boasted

250 big chunky stones on beautiful white silk taffeta with a skirt overlay. We built a special cage out of PVC tubing and wire from the hardware store, which my electrician wired with twelve sets of mini diamond-shaped lights powered by twelve AA batteries. The lights had to be sewn in by hand because we couldn't use a machine to sew electrical wire. The battery packs were sewn into pockets we created inside the cage. A giant snowflake headpiece was created to light up. It took eight of my staff four full days to complete.

Gel Hell

One of my seamstresses was sewing bra cups into a prom dress and didn't realize that the cups were filled with gel. She found out fast when the sewing-machine needle pierced the cup, sending gel oozing out and staining the dress. I immediately sent the dress out to be dry cleaned, and, although the stain wasn't entirely invisible, it was masked completely by stone embellishments adorning the bodice.

How Sweet It Is!

I once used 63 pounds of assorted candies to create a truly sweet sweet-sixteen dress for my TV show. I bought a colorful assortment of lollipops, gumballs, sourballs, jellybeans, candy sticks, rock candy, and paper strips of candy dots. Aqua and Light Turquoise crystals would add bling to the design. The short skirt and matching boned bustier were made with Tiffany-blue iridescent cellophane organza. A stiff petticoat of crinoline, wire, PVC tubing, and heavyweight interfacing provided stiff support for the candy-laden creation. The bustier was packed with candies in a delicious mosaic pattern. Accessories included heels packed with jelly beans and a lollipop "flower" accent, candy jewelry, and an elaborate headpiece. We used candy sticks, gummies, jellybeans, sourballs, gumballs, and lollipops, and, adding to the headpiece's crowning achievement, a tiny gumball machine that worked. But we didn't stop there. I was asked by the show's producers to make the dress emit a candy fragrance. I wired a small atomizer filled with cotton candy perfume to spray from the center front of the bodice. The spray pump was hidden in a pocket sewn into the interior lining of the skirt.

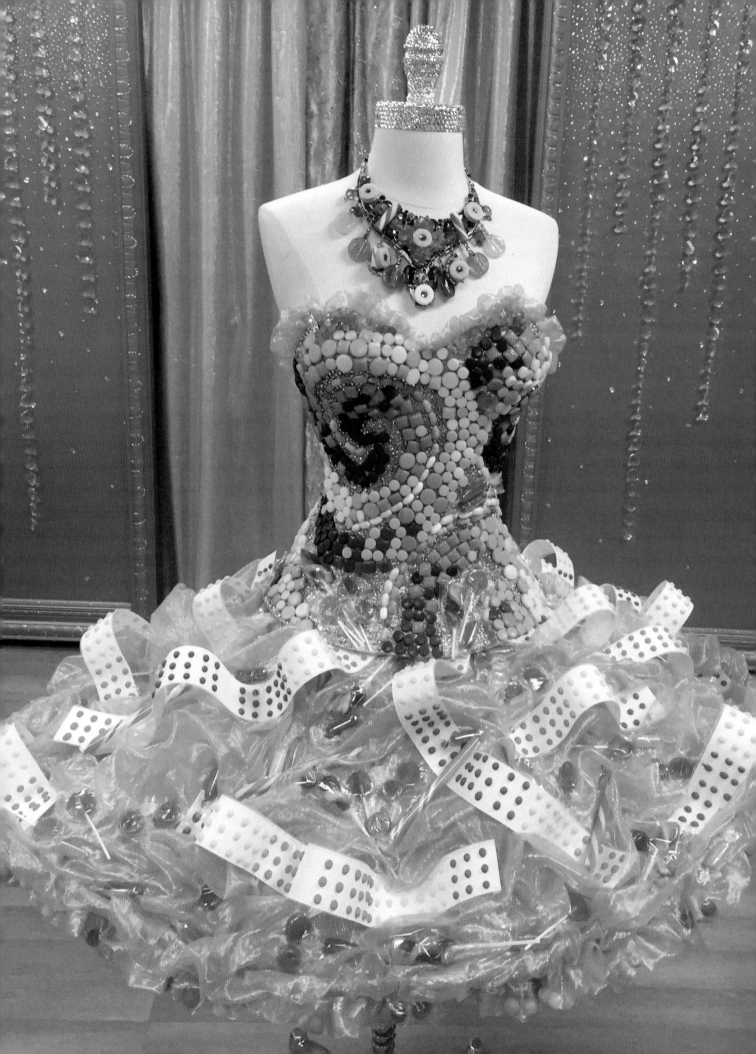

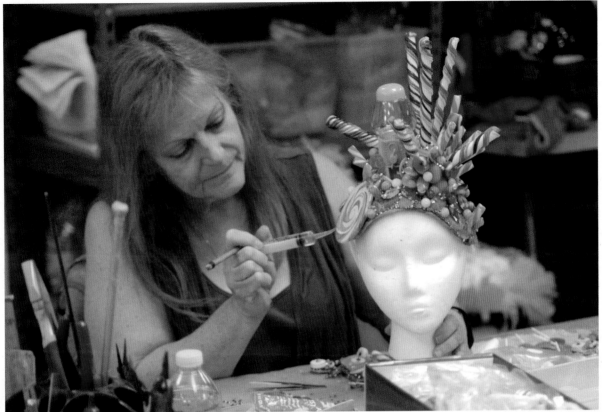

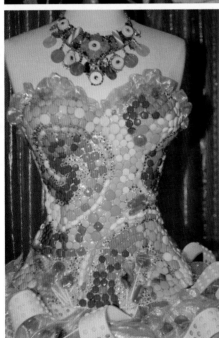

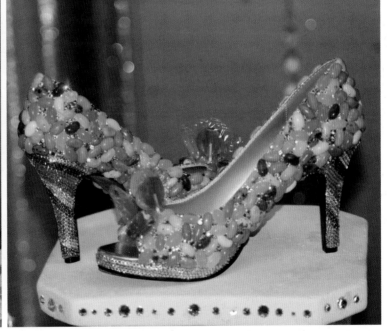

Above The crowning candy achievement was a custom headpiece featuring a working gumball machine! *Courtesy of Tisi Farrar*

Bottom left My Sweet 16 candy mosaic featured crystals and candies, including lollipops, sours, gumballs, jelly beans, and more! *Courtesy of Tisi Farrar*

Opposite How many types of candy can you find on this "taste-full" creation? *Courtesy of Tisi Farrar*

Bottom right The sweetest pair of heels you'll ever find. *Courtesy of Tisi Farrar*

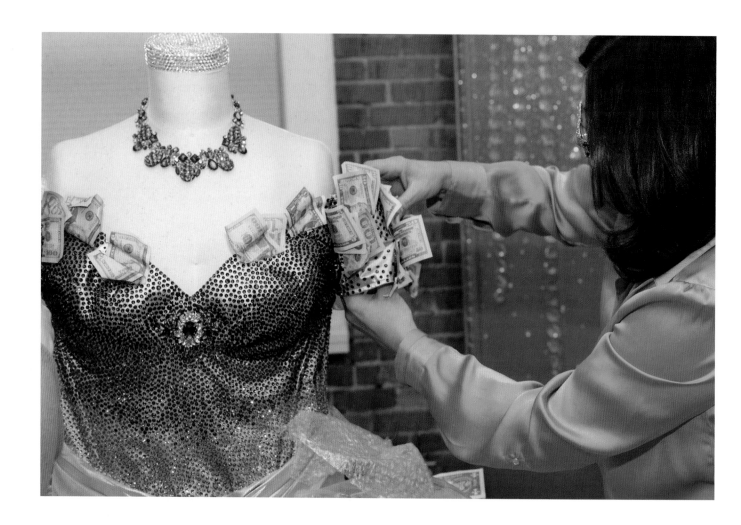

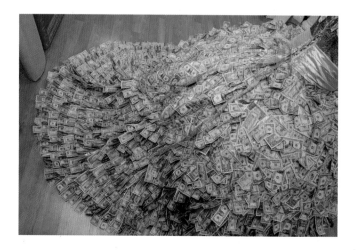

Now this is what I call a money train. (Can you spot the real bills?) *Courtesy of Tisi Farrar*

Top Think adding more money to the bustier makes "cents"? *Courtesy of Tisi Farrar*

Opposite top left Maria sews paper "money" onto gold lamé fabric to make the skirt. *Courtesy of Tisi Farrar*

Opposite top right Bouquet made using faux money folded into rosettes. *Courtesy of Tisi Farrar*

The Million-Dollar Dress

It was a first for me. The challenge was to custom design a dress made of money. I did some searching and found replica bills in assorted denominations and ordered 15,000 pieces. The fake cash was sewn onto panels of gold lamé that formed a large skirt. The skirt was supported by a custom hoop skirt and petticoat to add both fullness and support. The bodice had 8,800 Swarovski® crystals in the colors of Emerald, Fern, and Light Colorado. More replica bills were used to accent the neckline. In addition, several hundred real dollar bills were sewn into the design. The finishing touch to the ensemble was the custom bridal bouquet, made with handcrafted money roses, gold coins, gold satin ribbon, and gold-beaded mesh. If the replica bills used to create the dress had been genuine money, the ensemble would have been worth an estimated one million dollars!

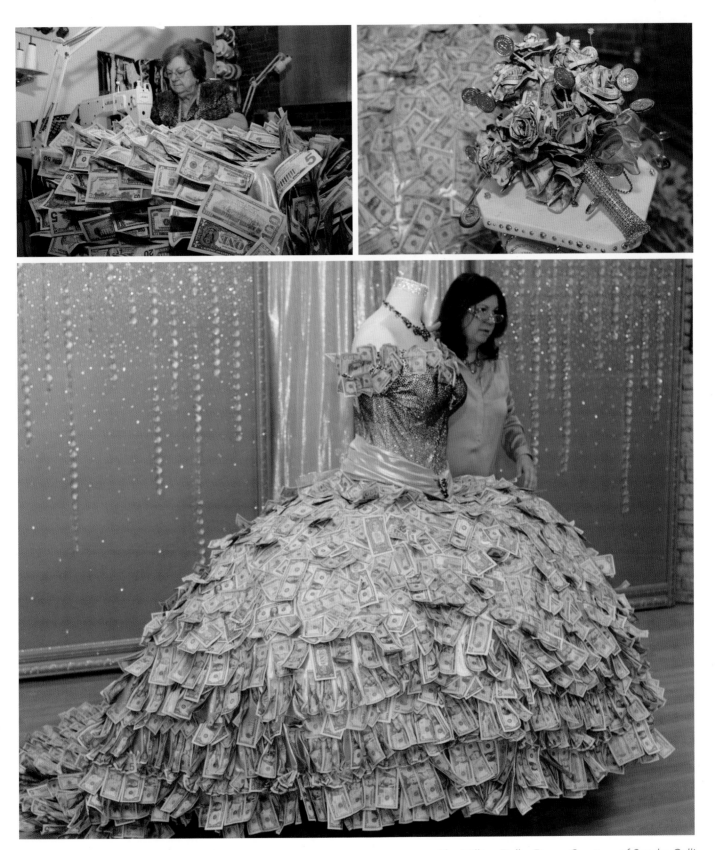

The Million-Dollar Dress. *Courtesy of Sondra Celli*

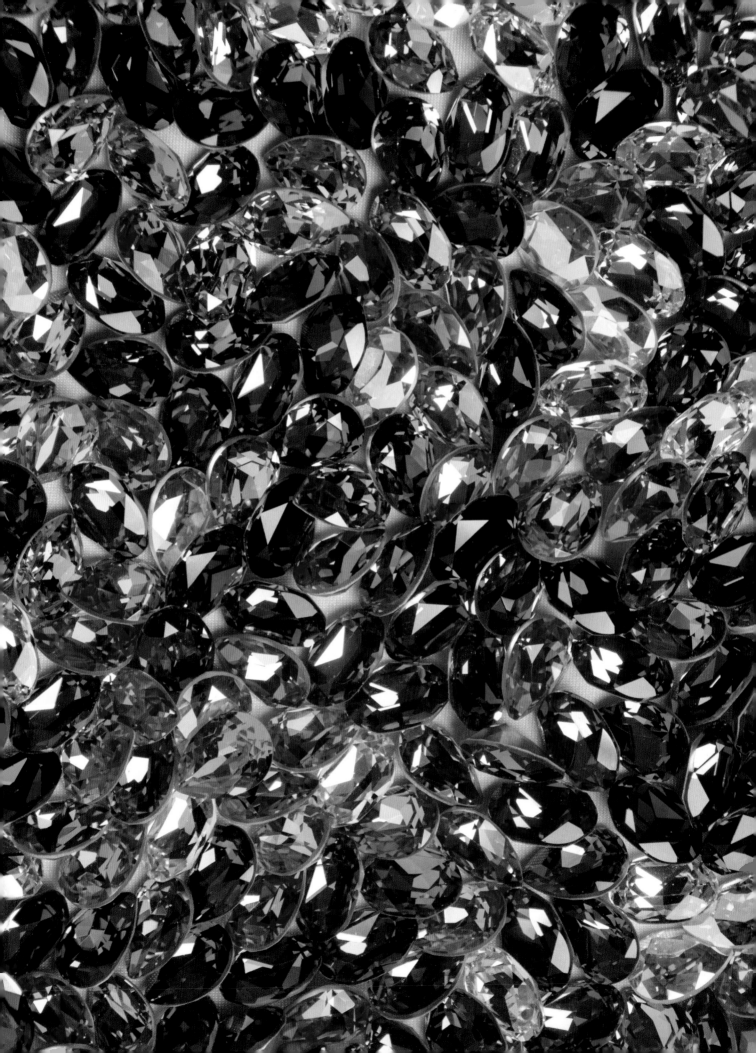

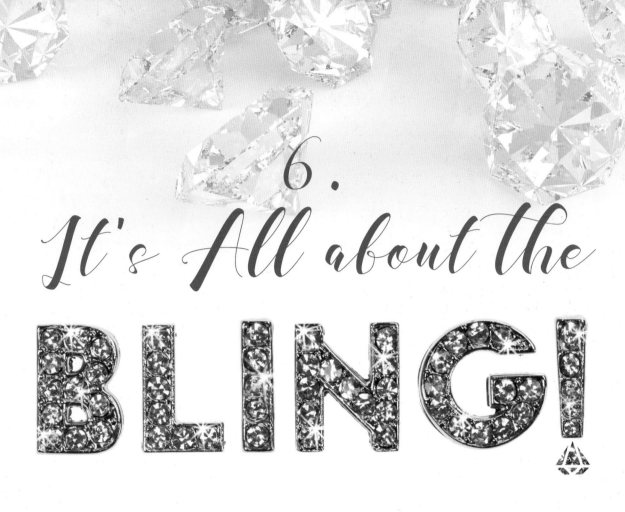

6.
It's All about the
BLING!

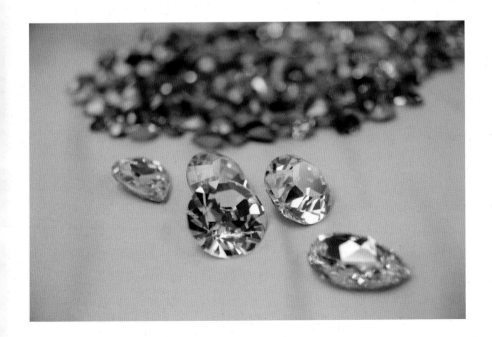

As almost everyone knows by now, I prefer to use genuine Swarovski® crystals for my custom couture because their sparkle is unmatched. You cannot find more-brilliant stones anywhere. They sparkle like diamonds and are as close to flawless as you can get. Compared to an ordinary crystal, Swarovski® has four times the facets, creating two and a half times the brilliance. The gleaming stones have been used as adornment for decades on gowns, accessories, chandeliers, costumes for the silver screen, and Broadway sets, and you might even have caught them glistening from atop New York City's Rockefeller Center Christmas Tree in the shape of a 550-pound star.

Due to their high quality, Swarovski® stones are expensive, but they are worth the price. The exquisite stones come in a wide variety of colors, shapes, and sizes. I love mixing them all together to create designs that are unique, textural, and multidimensional.

It's true that eye-catching bling can dramatically accentuate a design or transform something plain into attention-getting, which is one of the reasons bling is more mainstream than ever before. It is no longer relegated to bridal gowns and red carpet dresses–the stunning stones can be found on sneakers, jeans, athletic gear, pillows, eyeglasses, pet wear, and more.

My clients come in every age, shape, and size, and the vast majority of them request crystal embellishments. Those who don't want to go overboard will order lightly accented or trimmed items, while big fans of bling will lean toward the "pack 'em on" direction. Bling is in. From teen fashion rebels to fashionable moms and stylish seniors–millions of fans are addicted to those radiant rocks.

Embellishments

When my staff embellishes with stones, every pattern is drafted by hand first. Once the design is sketched out using a gel pen, the stones are methodically hand placed and adhered to the material. It's like painting with stones. For more-intricate or more-packed designs, I might assign six to eight of my staff to do the work. In addition to crystals, there are other varieties of bling that I love to work with. All the materials mentioned below can be sourced online at various craft or fabric stores. Here are some of my favorites, along with the pros and cons of working with each type.

Flat Backs

These are our basic stones that we use the most in the shop because they come in a wide variety of colors, shapes, and sizes. Flat backs also come in a hot-fix style, which you can apply with a hot-fix tool. These stones can be applied tightly together (packed) to make the most impressive effect. **Pro:** You have a wide variety of stones to choose from. **Con:** Patience is needed because intricate work is detailed and time-consuming.

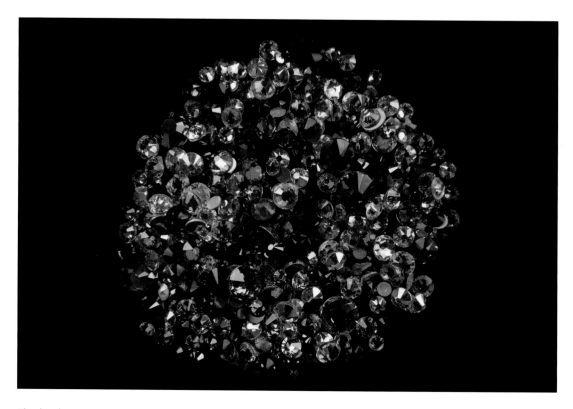

Flat backs.

Sew-On Jewels

These are flat-back stones with holes in them so that they can be sewn onto fabric. **Pro:** They come in wide variety of colors, shapes, and sizes. **Con:** Because they are heavy stones, they must be sewn on by hand, which can be time-consuming.

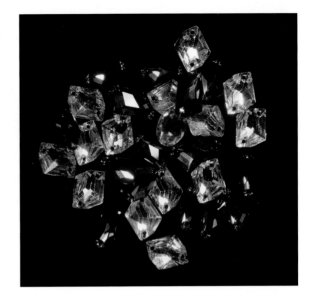

Sew-on jewels.

Fancy Stones with Settings

These are stones that are set in a silver or gold setting, secured by prongs. They have holes at the bottom and top of each setting so that you can sew the fancy stones onto fabric, or they can come without holes and you can just glue them onto fabric. **Pro:** Fancy stones give a gleaming 3-D effect to designs because they don't lie flat on fabric. **Con:** Setting the stones must be done by hand. It's a time-consuming process, using long-nosed pliers to bend the setting prongs over stones and tightly securing them in place. Also, prongs can sometimes catch on knit fabrics.

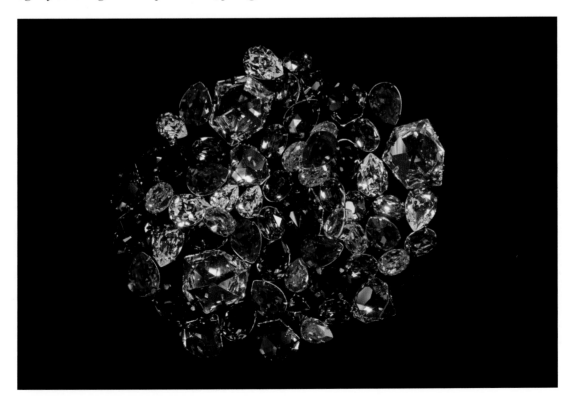

Fancy stones with settings.

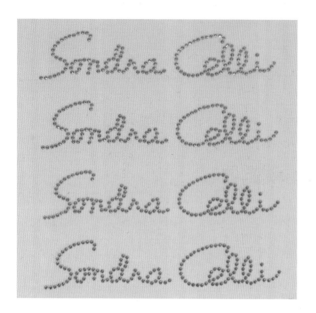

Heat-set transfers.

Heat-Set Transfers

These are premade crystal motifs that come on a piece of paper in various designs that you apply to fabric using heat, such as an iron. Heat-set transfers are good if you are a beginner "Bling-ette" or in a rush to finish a design. **Pro:** They come in a variety of premade designs and are a fast way to embellish. **Con:** If you don't use the correct heat setting, the stones will not adhere properly to fabrics.

Crystal Beads

These come in faceted shapes with a hole through the middle so that they can be sewn on. They can accompany any other types of crystal products to add a dramatic 3-D effect. **Pro:** Can be used to make intricate designs in very small areas. **Con:** Not as powerful if you are looking for shine. Faceted stones provide much more brilliance.

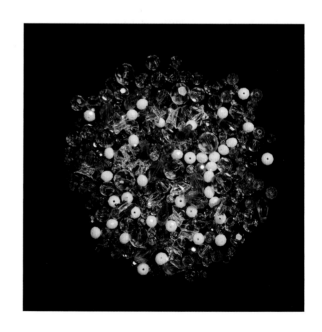

Crystal beads.

Crystal Cup-Chain Fringe

These are strands of cased crystals linked together in a chain form. **Pro:** Light reflects off the dangling crystals to provide sparkling movement when you walk or dance. **Con:** Cannot be used on knits or spandex because the chain catches on the fabric and leaves pulls.

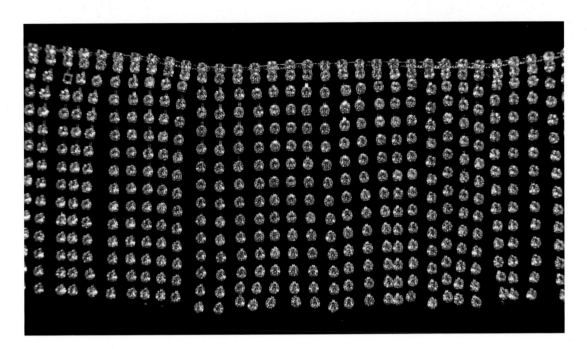

Crystal cup-chain fringe.

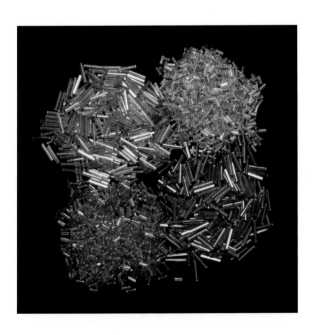

Bugle Beads

These are tubular beads that come in different lengths, sizes, and colors and can create a liquid beaded effect. They are usually made of glass or crystal. They are small and are sewn on to fabrics by hand. **Pro:** Can be mixed with crystals for more creative detail in a design. **Cons:** Bugle beads have more of a matte look to them, resulting in far less shine than crystals, and they can be time-consuming because they must be sewn on by hand.

Bugle beads.

Glass-Beaded Fringe

This is my favorite fringe, made up of tiny glass beads sewn together in strands–when light hits those beads, it's sparkle time. This kind of embellishment is great for adding movement to a design. **Pro:** Adding fringe turns simple designs into much more dynamic designs in no time. **Con:** The strip of ribbon that holds the fringe together should ideally be covered to blend in better with the fabric you are embellishing.

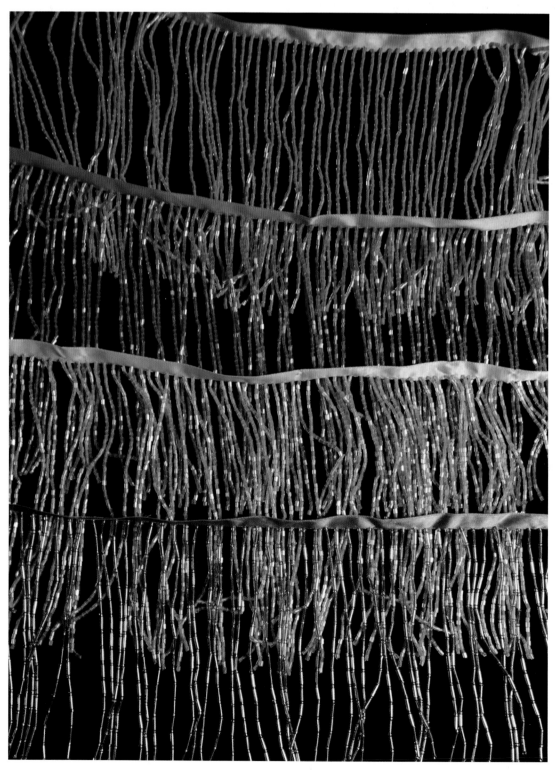

Glass-beaded fringe.

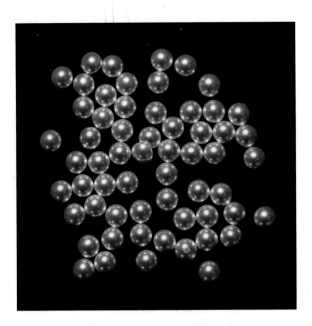

Flat-Back Pearls

A tried-and-true embellishment that never goes out of style. Swarovski® makes flat-back pearls in various colors to glue on. **Pro:** They can be glued on instead of sewn and provide a softer effect in design. **Con:** The muted effect of flat-back pearls can't compete with the brilliance of flat-back crystals. But they do pair well together when mixed into a design.

Flat-back pearls.

Jewelry Pieces

I like to take tiaras, necklaces, bracelets, earrings, pendants, and brooches and break them up into pieces to create visually stunning 3-D motifs. It looks terrific on a dress, bodice, shoe, or jacket. People who know me will often bring me old costume jewelry or unusual decorative pieces they find at flea markets or garage sales. The word on the street is to "bring it to Sondra, she'll make magic out of it." **Pro:** Building texture and dimension into a design is creatively exciting and innovative. **Con:** Designs must be carefully mapped out ahead of time. You don't want to just pile on and end up with a mess of metal remnants that turn your artistic, chic ready-to-wear into a clumsy "too heavy to wear."

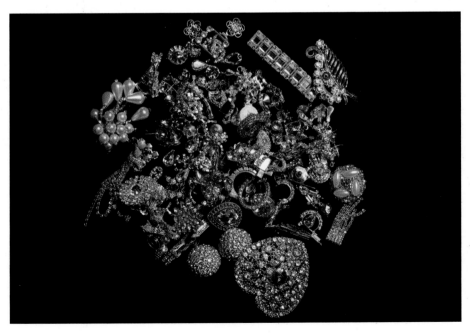

Jewelry pieces.

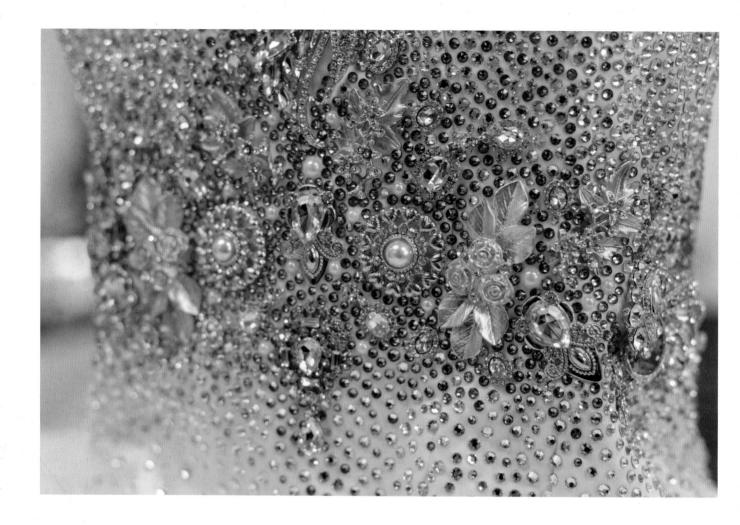

I absolutely avoid plastic stones because they look cheap and lack sparkle. They aren't bling; they are blah. Also, certain glues will eat through the plastic foil facing on the backs of plastic stones, causing them to cloud up.

Bling isn't the only way to embellish. When I was starting out as a designer, I used rhinestones but also worked a lot with feathers, ribbons, beading, silk flowers, and fringe to give designs that added wow factor. Fringe is great because there are so many types to choose from: leather, suede, fabric, chainette, etc., and it creates great movement in a design. When you move, it moves. If you want to cause a sensation, mixing crystals with fringe into a design will certainly do it. I rarely use sequins unless a client expressly requests them, since sequins are lackluster in comparison to the brilliance of crystals.

Assorted crystals and jewelry pieces combine to form a glistening bodice for a masquerade ball gown. *Courtesy of Mark Johnson*

All photos in this chapter courtesy of Mark Johnson

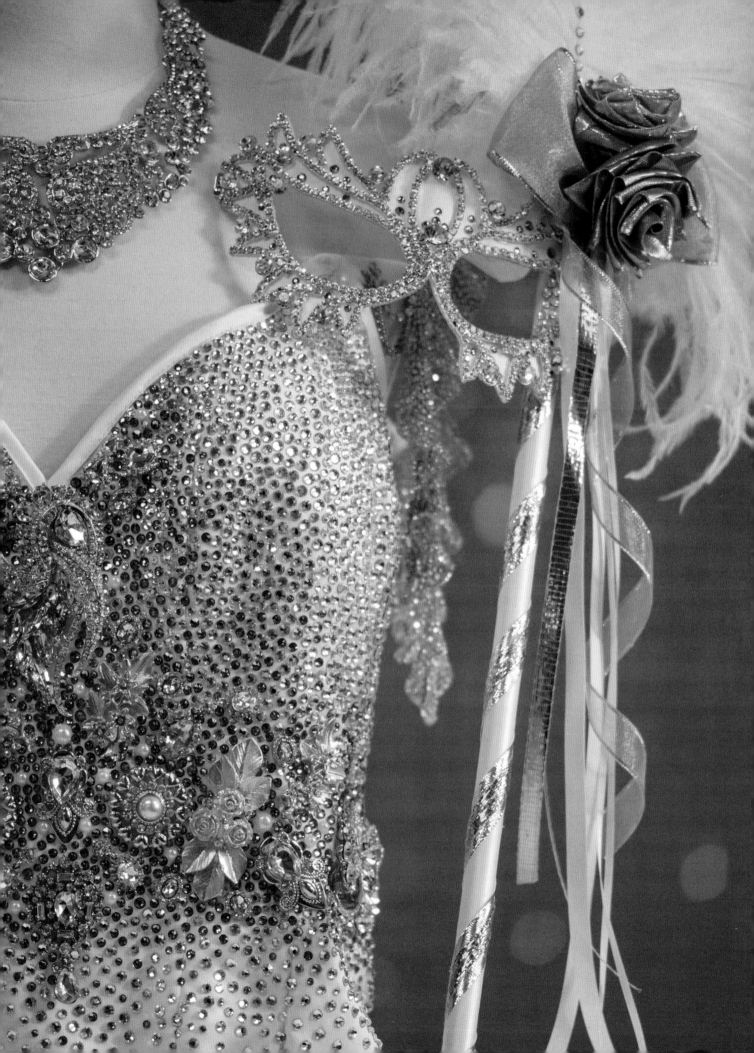

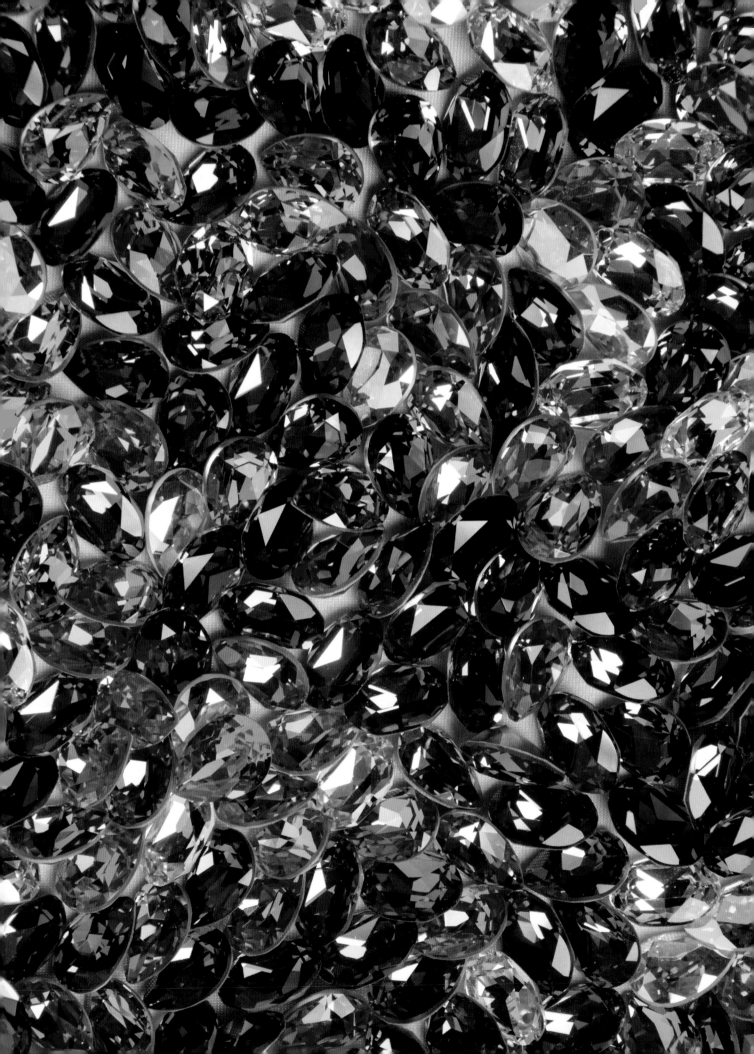

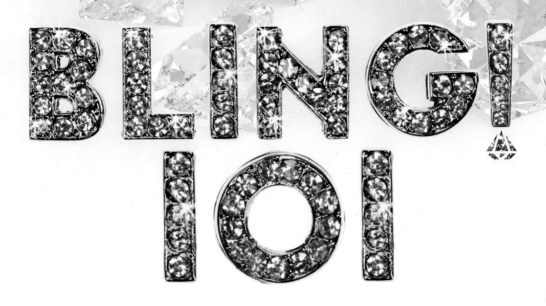

BLING! 101

7.
Getting Started

For years, fans of all ages and from all over the world have begged me to teach them how to bling. Let me now walk you through a variety of relatively easy bling projects that you can do at home. I'll take you step by step through each process. The finished embellished pieces can be added to your wardrobe or given as gifts. You will see how adding a few crystals to almost anything can transform it from basic blah to bling-tastic!

The seven techniques shared in this book are the same ones we use in my shop. I suggest reading through the instructions once or twice before starting any project. Also, give yourself time to really learn the basics. Once you have those down, you can get as creative as you want. There are no limits to what you can do with a few sparkling stones and a little bit of solid know-how.

Materials
You Will Need

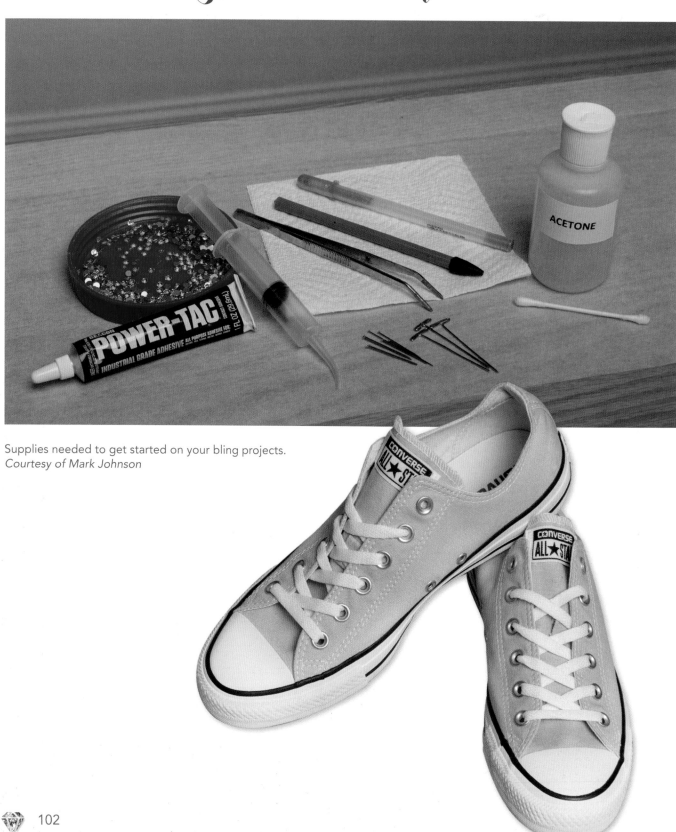

Supplies needed to get started on your bling projects.
Courtesy of Mark Johnson

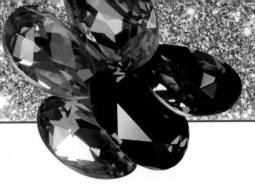

Before beginning any project, make sure to have all your materials on hand.
Here is what you'll need:

Item you wish to bling

Parchment paper

Gel pen

Glue (Power-Tac®)

Crystals

Shallow container

Bling tool

Syringe

Straight pins or T-pins

(for the Ombré and Floral and Swirl techniques, as well as cleanup)

Paper towels

Long-handled tweezers

Cotton swabs

Acetone

After you've gathered all your materials together, follow the guidelines below.

Guidelines for Getting Started

Let's go through a few basics of the process. There are three main parts to your project:

SETUP, CLEANUP, AND REVIEW.

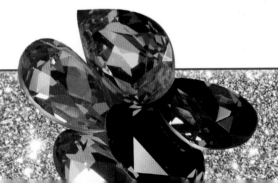

Setup

Create a clean work space at a desk or work table in a room providing great light and ventilation. Protect the top of your work service by covering it with parchment paper. As you choose and use the other materials, keep these tips in mind.

Gel Pen

You may find it helpful to plan your design in advance to know where you will place the crystals. If that is the case, you can use a gel pen to lightly mark areas with small dots showing placement of the crystals. We suggest using a silver-colored gel pen because the ink is light and barely noticeable. Dots should be small enough to be covered by the stones once you glue them down.

Glue

There are many adhesives on the market today to choose from, but we recommend POWER-TAC®. It has very little odor, dries clear, and, if used properly, adheres crystals to most fabrics. It is included in my Sondra Celli Bling Kit, available at www.beaconadhesives.com/blingkit.

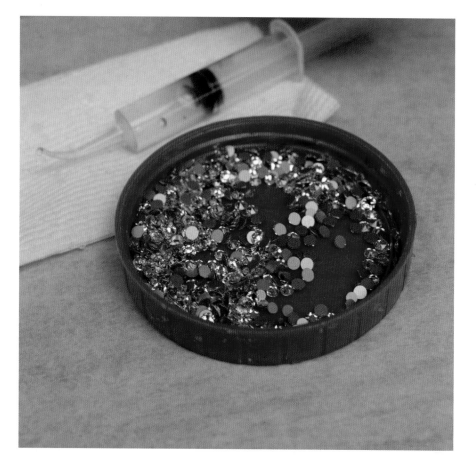

Crystals

As a general rule, Clear is a basic Swarovski® crystal color that resembles ice. It works well no matter what you are embellishing because it complements all colors. As for the size of the crystals, we use a variety, depending on the project. For more-intricate designs, we use the tiny 5ss (stone size) to 10ss. These are harder to work with and best left to more-expert DIY bling enthusiasts. We also use larger stones (20ss and up), but when you use bigger crystals you'll limit the number of everyday objects you can bling. The majority of our custom designs are embellished with size 16ss stones, which we recommend for every one of the projects featured in this book. It is a medium-sized stone and much easier to work with if you are a novice.

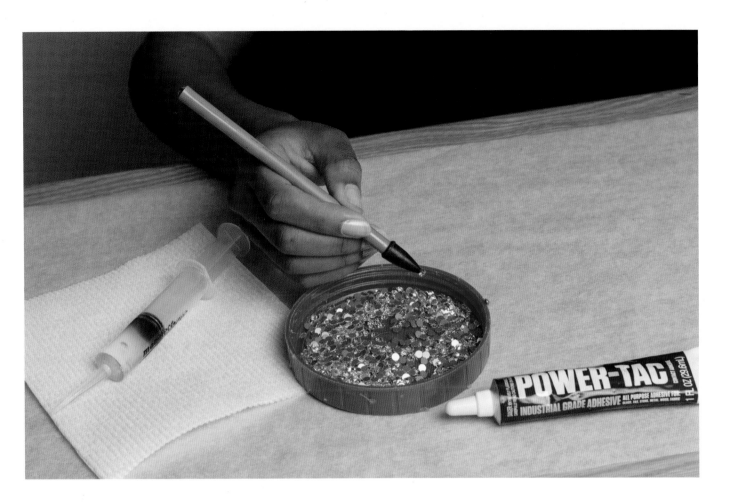

Shallow Container

Use a wide, shallow container to hold your crystals. This makes it much easier to access the stones and pick them up by using the bling tool.

Bling Tool

The bling tool's waxy tip makes picking up crystals easy. Pick up crystals one at a time by the top, shiny, faceted side. Place a crystal on the glue (flat side down) and lightly, but firmly, press the crystal onto the fabric or item you are blinging. Note: With use, the bling tool's tip may flatten. To reshape tip back into a point, just roll the tip back and forth between your thumb and index finger while applying a bit of pressure. You can purchase a bling tool at www.beaconadhesives.com/blingkit either separately or as part of my Sondra Celli Bling Kit.

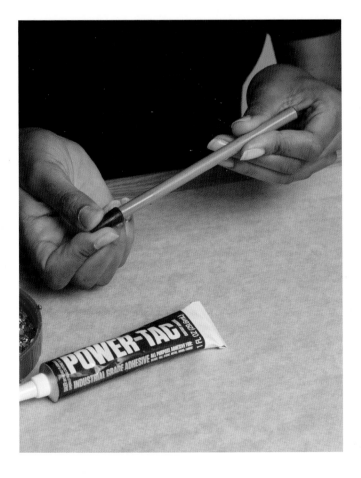

The bling tool can be easily reshaped.

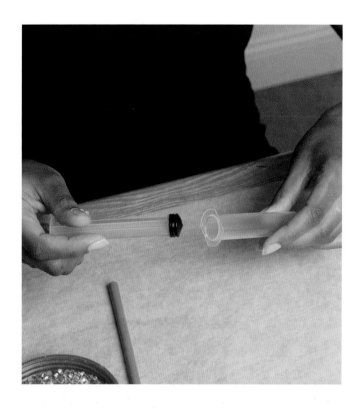

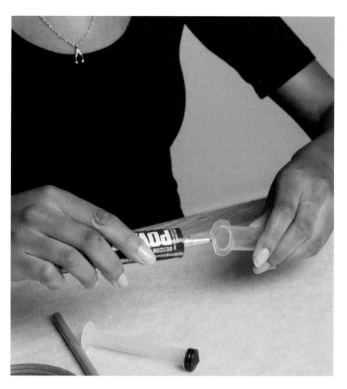

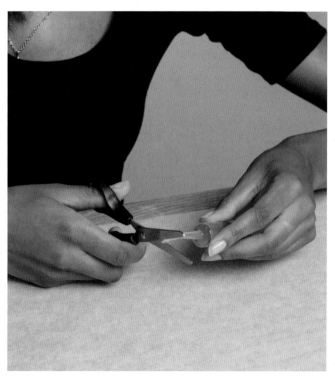

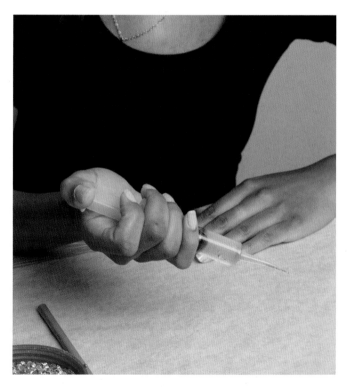

Syringe

Syringes can be sourced online or at www.amazon.com and are a great way to apply glue. Pull the plunger out of the syringe barrel and carefully squeeze glue into the barrel while holding the syringe at a 45-degree angle. Allow the glue to run slowly down the interior side of the barrel to prevent air bubbles from forming. Fill the syringe about a quarter of the way up with glue. You can always add more adhesive, but start with less so as not to waste glue.

Carefully insert the syringe plunger back into the barrel. Cut off the tip of syringe at an angle for easy flow. Test the flow by slowly pressing down on the plunger with your thumb until glue begins to ooze out from the tip. Wipe the tip clean and then try creating a series of glue "dots" to get used to the right amount of pressure you will need to make the dots small enough to be covered by crystals once you start blinging.

Straight or T-pins

These are needed for the ombré technique to indicate where you want to begin the transition from one tone into another and for the Floral and Swirl techniques to secure the pattern in place while you trace the design onto the fabric. Straight or T-pins are also used for cleanup to clear away any dried glue from the syringe tip.

Paper Towels

Use this to wipe away any excess glue from the tip of the syringe before using. You want to control the amount of adhesive you are applying to avoid drowning your crystals in glue or staining the fabric. You'll also use paper towels to clean the syringe when you have finished with your project ("Cleanup" below).

Long-Handled Tweezers

Use tweezers to peel away dried glue that has accumulated in the barrel of the syringe.

Cotton Swabs

For cleanup. If needed, moisten a cotton swab with acetone to clean stones of excess dried glue and to remove any residual wax left by the bling tool after your project is finished (see "Review" below).

Acetone

Use sparingly for cleaning up stones. Make sure cotton swab is moistened and not soaked with acetone.

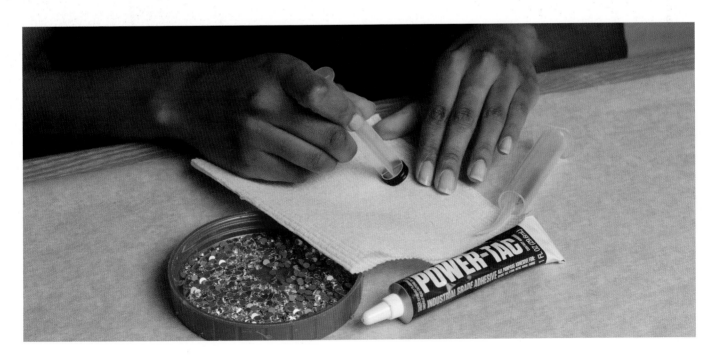

Use a paper towel to remove all glue from syringe plunger and barrel.

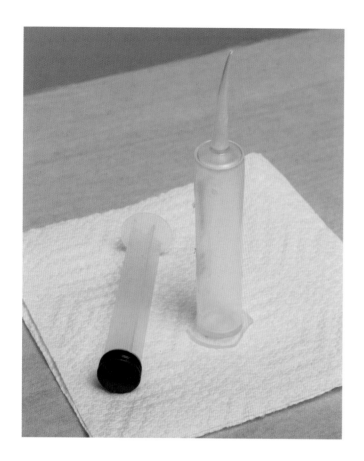

Left Leave syringe to air-dry overnight in two pieces set on a paper towel. Barrel should be inverted so that any tiny traces of adhesive will drain onto the towel.

Below A T-pin can help clear the syringe tip of any dried adhesive.

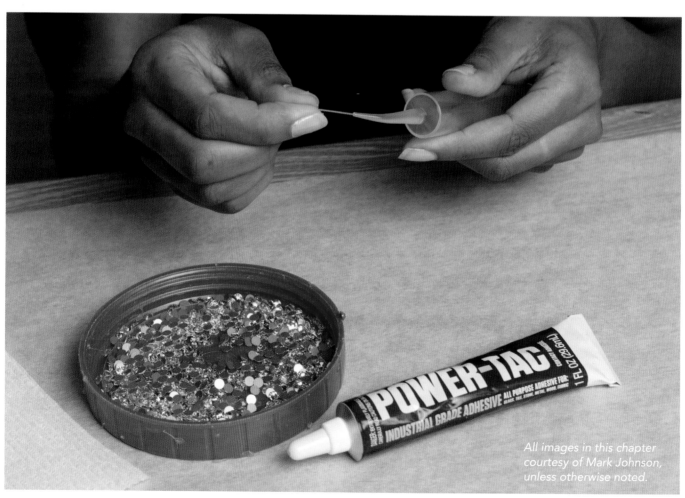

All images in this chapter courtesy of Mark Johnson, unless otherwise noted.

Cleanup

When you have finished your project, squeeze any remaining adhesive from the syringe into a paper towel. Pull syringe apart and wipe away excess glue from the plunger and interior barrel of the syringe. Allow syringe to dry overnight in two separate pieces. Barrel should drain dry on a paper towel, with the tip pointing up. The next day, use tweezers to peel away any remaining dried glue from the barrel interior and a T-pin to clean out the syringe tip. After the syringe is cleaned, it can be used again for your next bling project.

Review

Once your bling project is finished and completely dried (allow a full twenty-four hours), review your work. Look for any waxy residue that may be left on stones from the bling tool. If there is some, dampen a cotton swab very lightly with acetone and gently wipe away. Do not soak the cotton swab with the acetone or you may ruin the fabric or the crystal's finish.

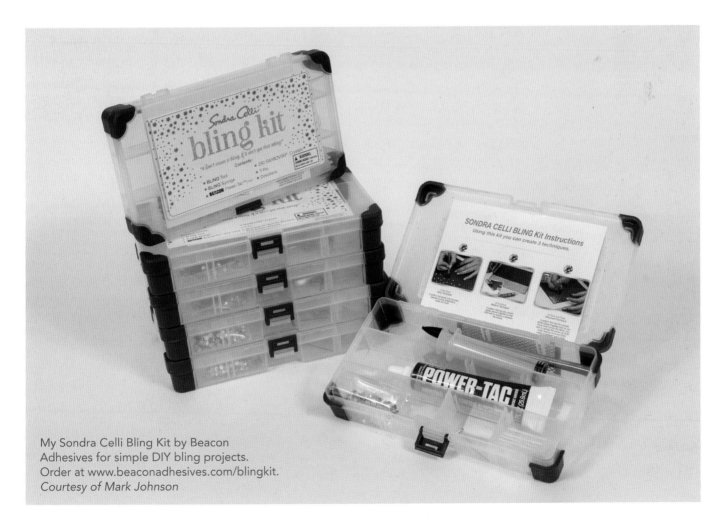

My Sondra Celli Bling Kit by Beacon
Adhesives for simple DIY bling projects.
Order at www.beaconadhesives.com/blingkit.
Courtesy of Mark Johnson

One last quick note about the adhesive I recommend for the projects in this book. It is imperative to use glue strong enough to bond crystals–especially to fabrics. My choice is POWER-TAC®. It is an all-purpose adhesive for most fabrics, glass, metal, wood, tile, and stone. Over the years I heard from countless do-it-yourselfers who complained about glues that didn't hold the stones or were too messy to work with. I decided to find a solution to the problem and teamed up with Beacon Adhesives, a family-owned and family-operated business that has been producing adhesives in the industrial and craft industries for decades. POWER-TAC® is manufactured right here in the US and can be found in most craft stores.

In addition to POWER-TAC®, we designed a Sondra Celli Bling Kit for those wanting to learn how to embellish with bling. Each kit includes a 1-ounce tube of POWER-TAC®, 250 Clear crystals (size 16ss), a bling tool, a T-pin, a syringe, and instructions.

As a Thank you

For purchasing this book, we are offering a special discount on the bling kits. Place your order at www.beaconadhesives.com/ blingkit or just scan this QR code. Then use the code SCBOOK at checkout. This special code will be effective only for as long as supplies last.

8.
Dot Pack Technique

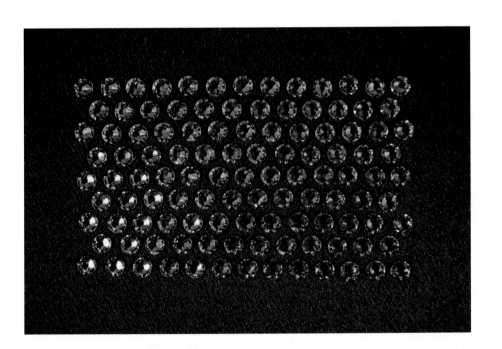

Example of the loose Dot Pack motif.

overwhelm it. A tight dot pack motif leaves less space in between the stones and gives any design a much more powerful impact.

Notice in the photo (left) how each row of stones builds upon the other by centering the stones in a pyramid formation. For example, look at the placement of the stone in the center of the top row. Now look at the placement of stones in the second row, directly below it. Notice the triangle? One stone on top and two stones directly below so that one is on the left and one on the right. Row 3 mimics the placement of the first stone in row 1. This works horizontally as well as vertically. Stacking stones in this manner, while leaving space in between, is called a loose Dot Pack technique. A tight Dot Pack technique leaves less space in between the stones. Refer to the sample photo above to help guide you with stone placement as you work.

There are two versions of the Dot Pack technique: loose and tight. A loose dot pack leaves space in between the crystals. The key to a perfect loose dot pack is to make sure the stones are placed with an equal amount of space in between each one. It's a great way to lightly add embellishment to a design or accessory but not

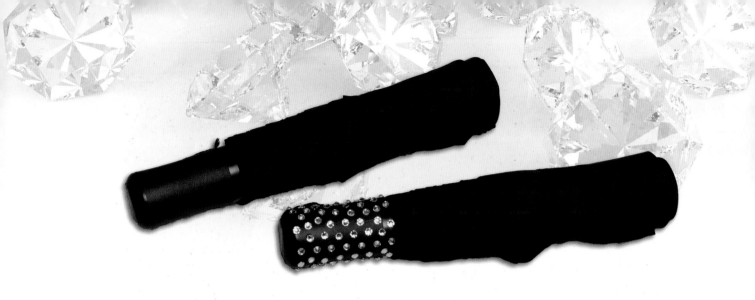

BLING–*Accented Umbrella*

Since the loose dot pack is one of the easiest bling techniques for beginners to learn, and since most people own an umbrella, we'll start here with our very first bling project. Don't worry about exact stone placement. As with everything, you'll get better with practice.

Review the list of "Materials You Will Need" and the "Getting Started" guidelines in chapter 7 (page 103) before beginning any project.

Above Shine even when it is raining with this bling-accented umbrella. It takes only a handful of crystals.

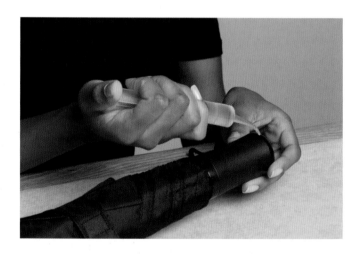

1

Using the glue-filled syringe, create a glue dot on the umbrella handle.

2

With the bling tool, pick up a stone (faceted side up) and place it onto the glue dot you just created. Press down lightly to secure its placement.

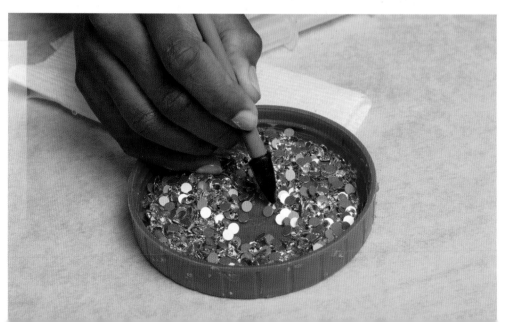

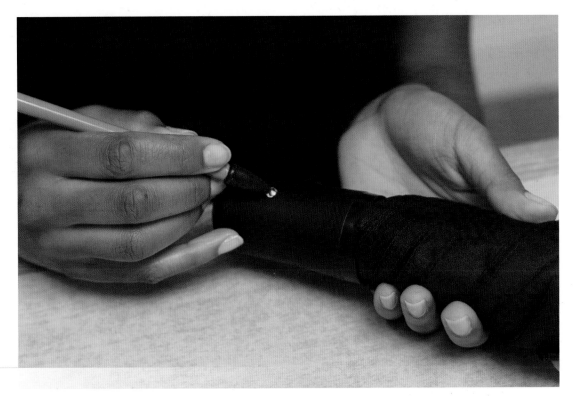

3 Leaving a small amount of space in between, create another glue dot and place another crystal below the first stone.

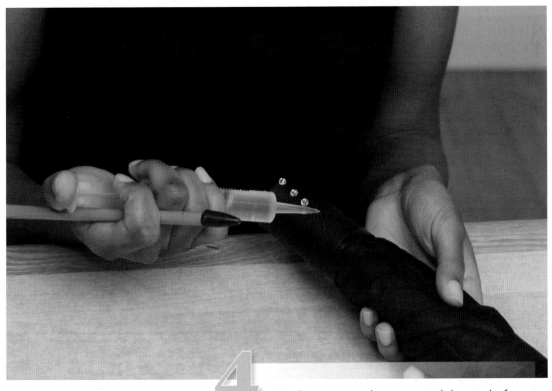

4 Work your way down toward the end of the umbrella handle, making a straight row of stones. Try to keep an equal amount of space in between the stones as you go.

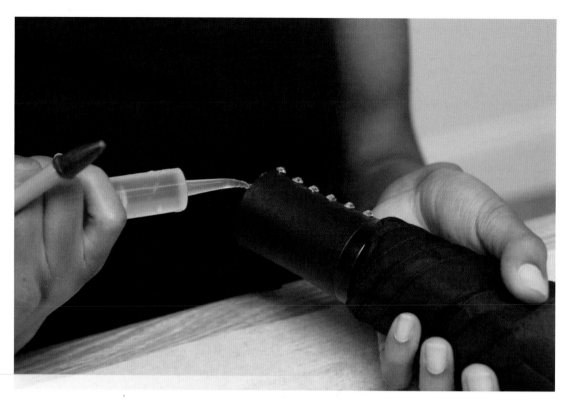

5 Now begin a new row of stones parallel to your first row in the same manner. Line up the stones in your second row to fit in the empty spaces between stones of the first row. Create a glue dot, place stone on the dot, leave a bit of space, and repeat.

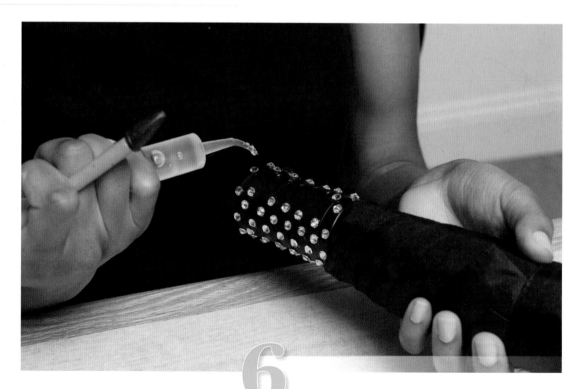

6 Continue creating straight rows of loosely packed stones parallel to the previous rows until handle has been entirely dot packed.

114

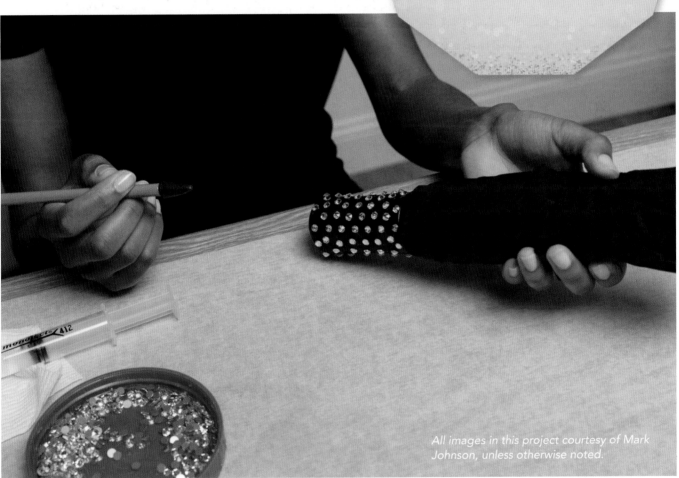

All images in this project courtesy of Mark Johnson, unless otherwise noted.

7

Allow umbrella to dry completely—a full twenty-four hours.

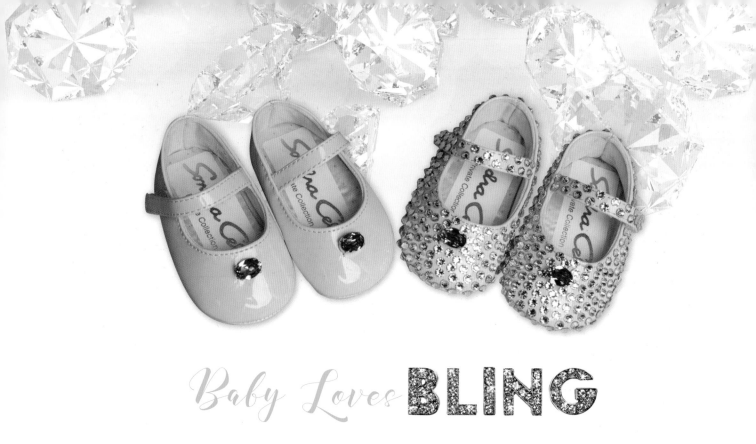

Baby Loves BLING

We'll continue taking baby steps with these easy bling projects until you become more comfortable with the process.

After my bling glasses, the most requested accessory is probably the blinged-out baby shoes. Clients buy them to announce a birth, for baptisms, and for birthdays. They also make cute Christmas tree ornaments!

Above Baby loves bling! *Courtesy of Mark Johnson*

Review the list of "Materials You Will Need" and the "Getting Started" guidelines in chapter 7 (page 103) before beginning any project.

1 We start this project by gluing a large accent stone to the top of the baby shoe. You could also use a tiny flower or bow instead.

2 Now move to the seam at the shoe sole and create a few tiny glue dots along the seam. Leave a little space in between each dot. Avoid using too much glue since the adhesive can ooze up onto the faceted face of the stones, inhibiting their shine.

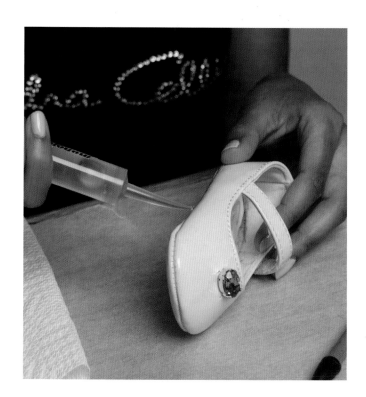

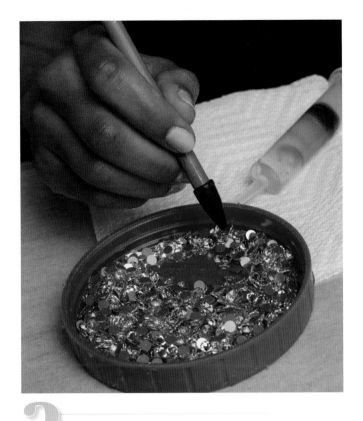

3 Pick up a crystal with the bling tool (faceted side up).

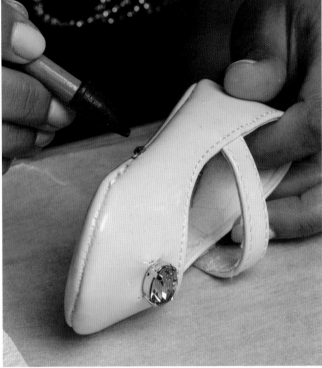

4 Gently press the stone onto the glue dot to secure it in place.

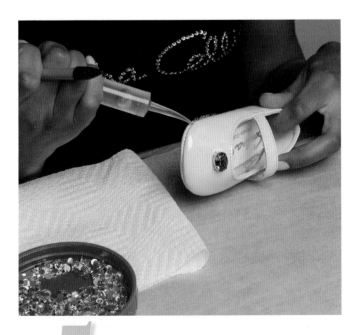

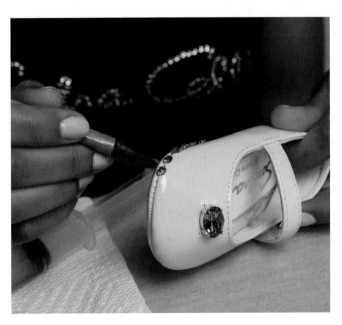

5 Continue applying glue dots and placing crystals on them along the seam of the shoe sole until it has been entirely outlined with stones.

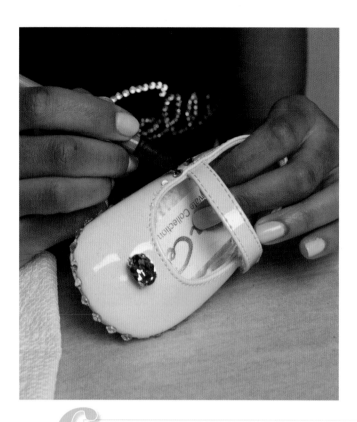
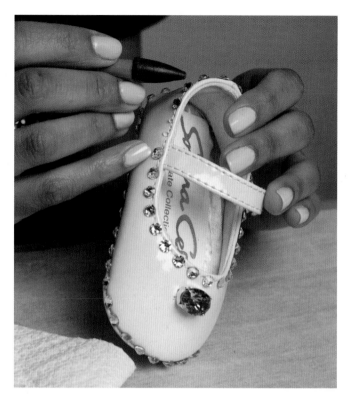

6 Once you finish stoning the sole seam, begin stoning the top edge of the shoe until it has been entirely outlined.

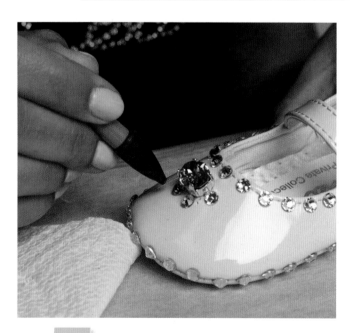
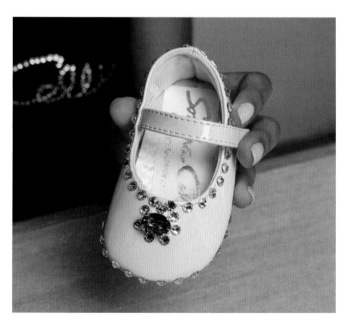

7 You always want to outline your project first before filling it in with stones. Outline the large accent stone with bling, leaving space in between the stones.

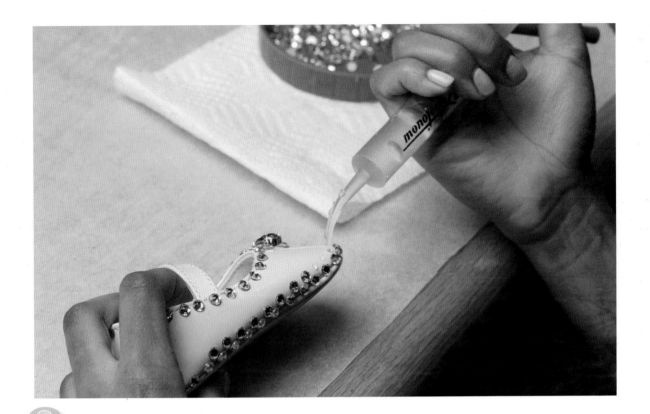

8

Now fill in the entire shoe with stones. Start by adding a row of stones above the first row you completed along the seam of the shoe sole and work up.

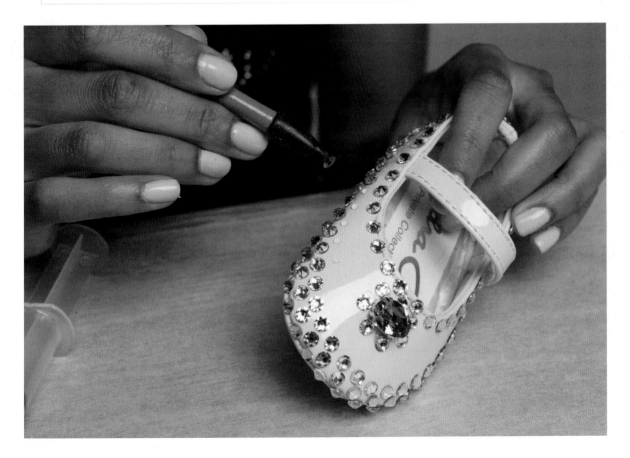

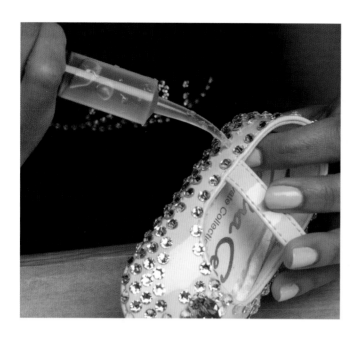
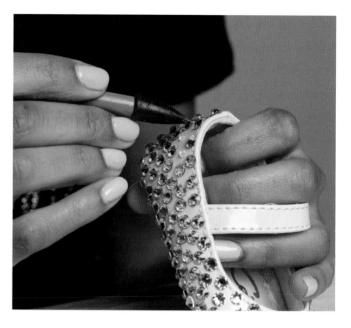

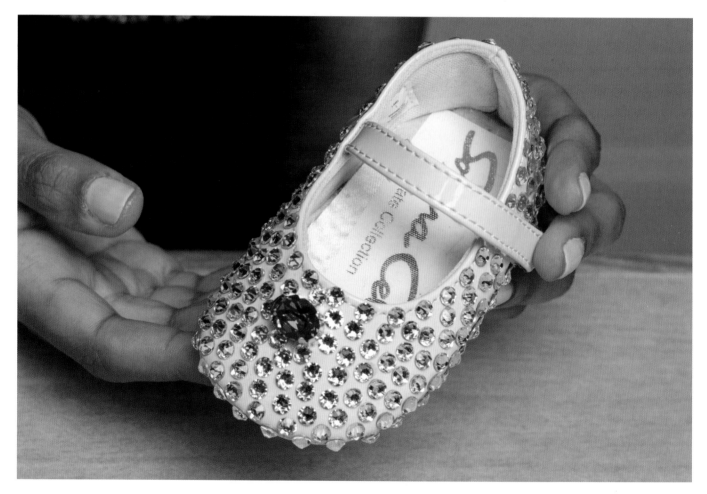

9

Continue adding rows one on top of the other until the shoe is covered with loosely packed stones.

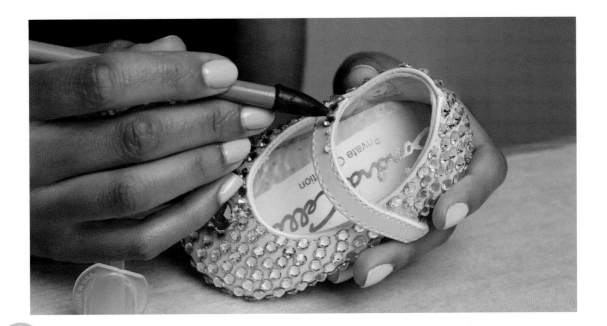

10

Now begin working across the top of the shoe strap with a row of stones.

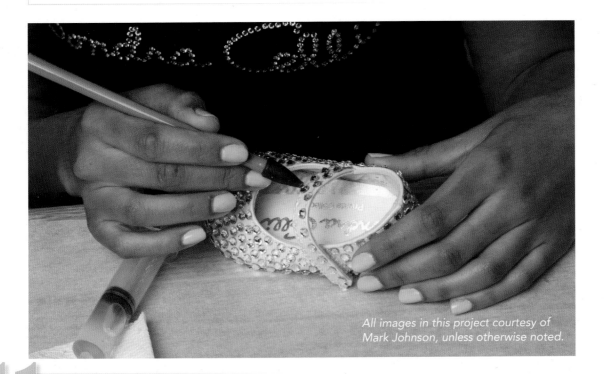

All images in this project courtesy of Mark Johnson, unless otherwise noted.

11

Finish by gluing a second row of stones across the shoe strap beneath the one you just completed.

12

Allow baby shoes to dry completely overnight.

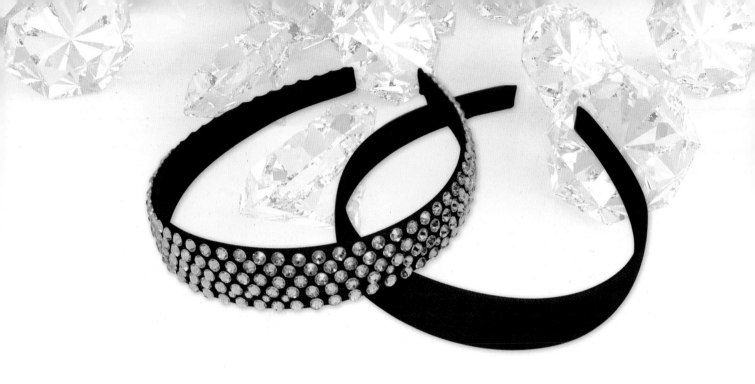

Head-Turning Headband

Use your head to embellish your wardrobe! Bling out a plain headband with stones by using the easy Dot Pack technique, and give your casual look more of an impact.

Review the list of "Materials You Will Need" and the "Getting Started" guidelines in chapter 7 (page 103) before beginning any project.

1 Begin by making a few small glue dots along the top edge of a headband. You can use either a fabric or plastic headband for this project.

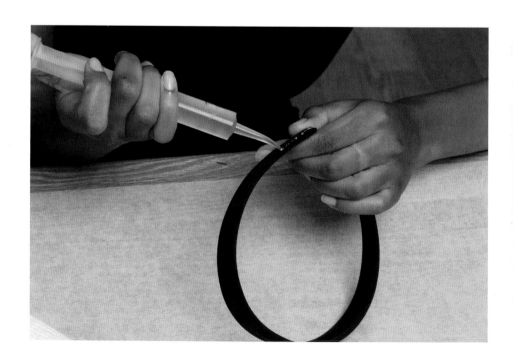

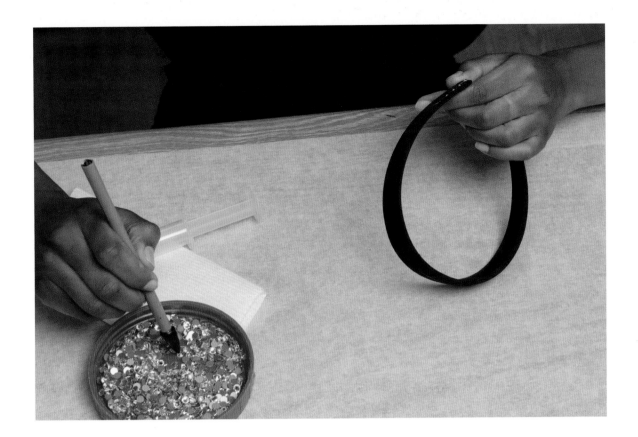

2 Picking up one stone at a time with your bling tool faceted side up, lightly press the stone down onto the glue dot. Continue gluing stones along the edge of the headband in a row. Leave a small amount of space in between each stone.

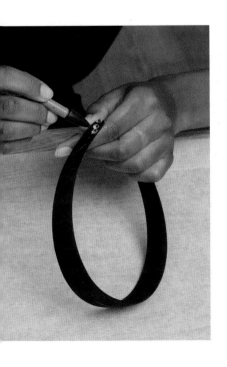
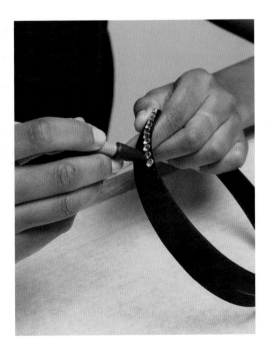
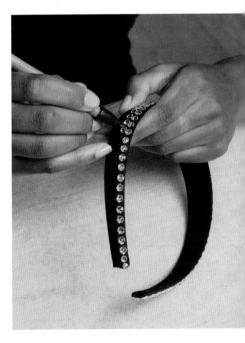

3

Once you have completed the first row, begin a new row directly below it in the same manner. Continue creating rows until the headband has been packed with stones.

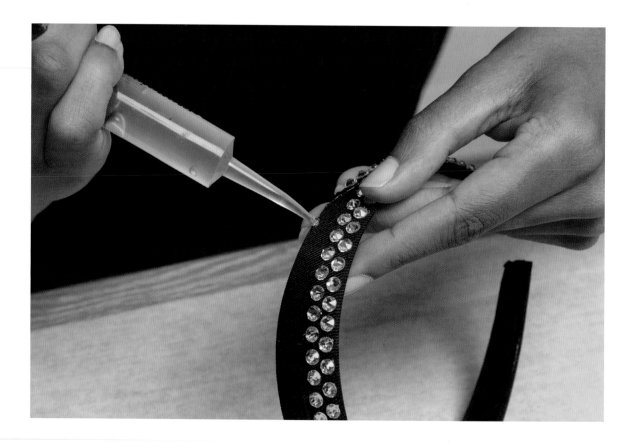

4

Allow headband to dry completely overnight.

Congratulations on your first three bling projects! Are you ready for more adventures in bling? We're moving on to our next technique– Interlock.

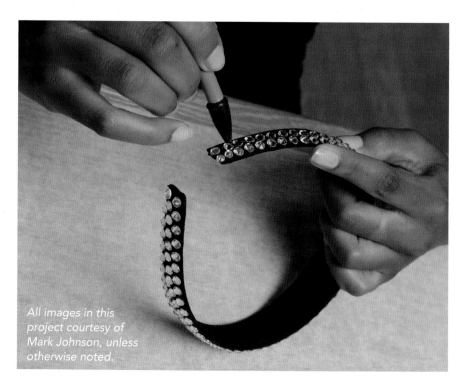

All images in this project courtesy of Mark Johnson, unless otherwise noted.

9.
Interlock Technique

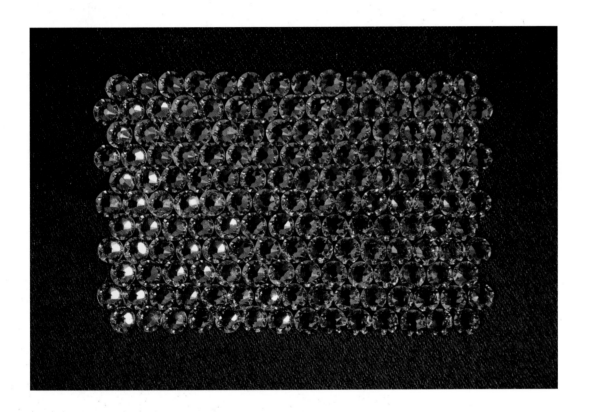

With the Interlock technique, crystals are glued so closely together that they are locked into place. When you use this technique, it's helpful to begin your project by outlining the surface area you want to bling first and then filling the area in with stones.

It gives a visually impressive result that truly packs a punch. If you want to be noticed, the Interlock technique is the way to go.

Example of the Interlock technique.

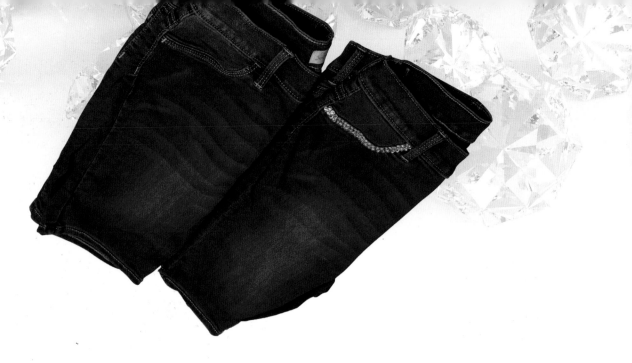

Hot Pockets

A pair of denim shorts is a great article to learn on because you can follow the stitching when embellishing with stones. For our demonstration we will keep it simple by highlighting just the front pockets of the shorts. If you want to add more bling, you can embellish along the waistband, belt loops, side seams, and pant hem. Refer to the sample Interlock technique photo above to help guide you with stone placement as you work.

Review the list of "Materials You Will Need" and the "Getting Started" guidelines in chapter 7 (page 103) before beginning any project.

Above Check out these denim shorts with just a touch of sparkling highlights. *Courtesy of Mark Johnson*

1 Begin by applying a very thin line of glue along the pocket stitching about an inch or two in length. You want just enough glue applied so that the crystals will cover it, yet won't ooze up and cover the stones.

2 Using the bling tool, apply the stones one by one to the line of glue, making sure that when you place the stones they are touching and tightly interlocked together. There should not be any space in between the stones.

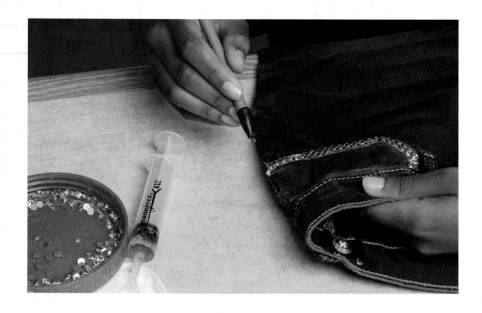

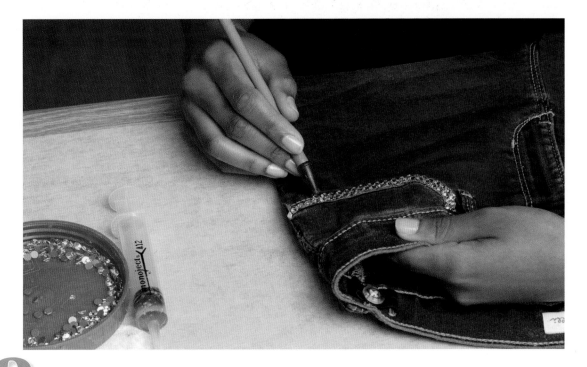

3 Once you have finished lining the top of the pocket, create a second row directly underneath in the same manner, tightly interlocking the stones.

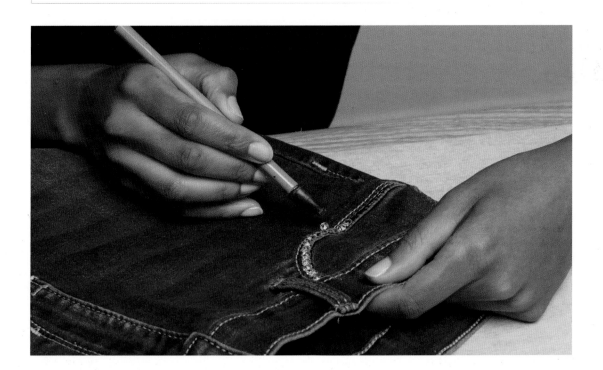

4 Now do the same thing to the other pocket. Apply a thin line of glue, following the pocket stitching. Using the bling tool, add stones to the glue, tightly locking them together as you go.

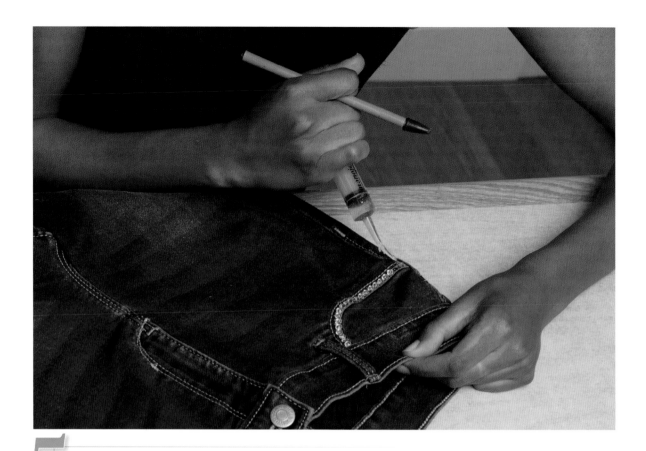

5 Begin gluing a second row of stones directly underneath the first.

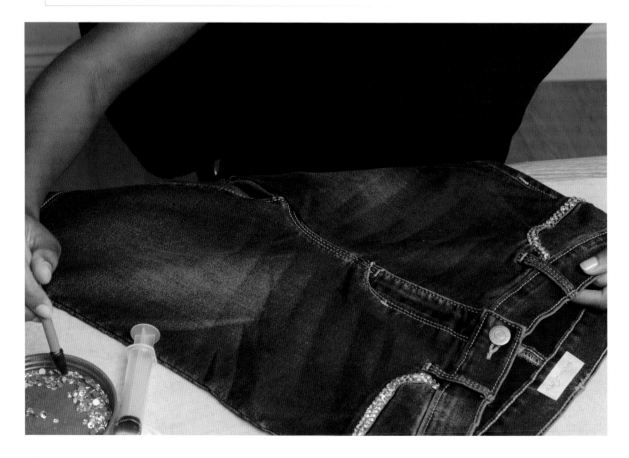

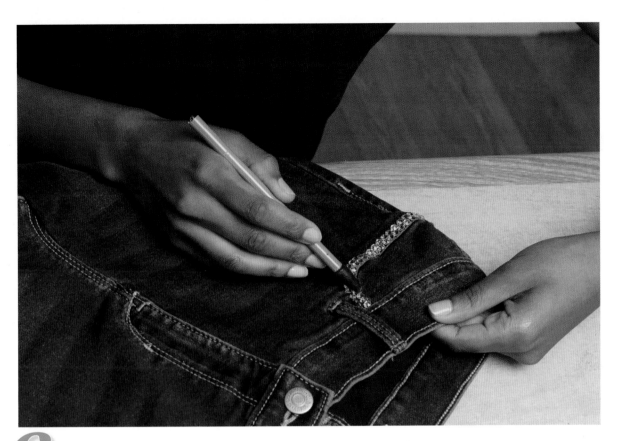

6 Allow shorts to dry completely overnight.

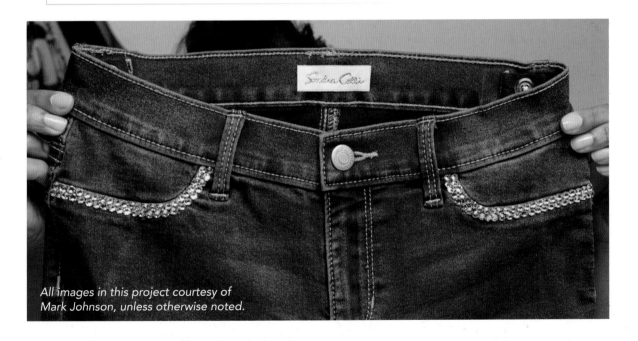

All images in this project courtesy of Mark Johnson, unless otherwise noted.

See how easy it is to add bling to your wardrobe?

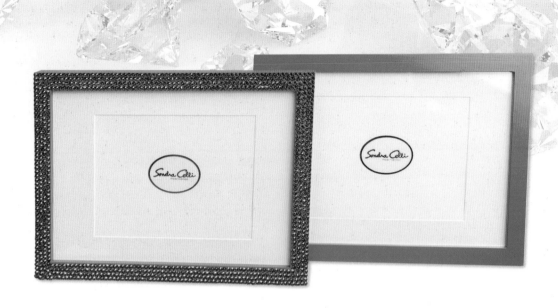

Picture Perfect

It's picture perfect! Adding bling to a frame makes a great engagement or bridal gift, or a special keepsake for any memorable event or cherished moment you want to preserve.

Review the list of "Materials You Will Need" and the "Getting Started" guidelines in chapter 7 before beginning any project.

1 Select a picture frame with a smooth, flat surface.

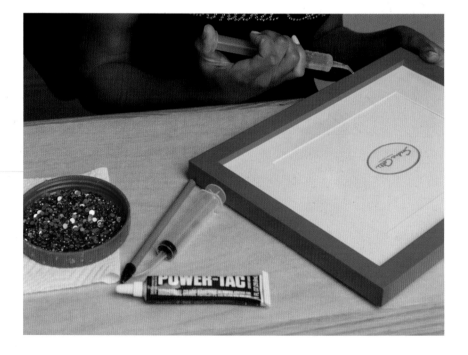

2 Starting on the outside edge of the frame, use the syringe to apply a thin line of glue. Apply only an inch or two of glue at a time, since it's more manageable to work with. As you become more comfortable and faster, you can work longer areas at a time.

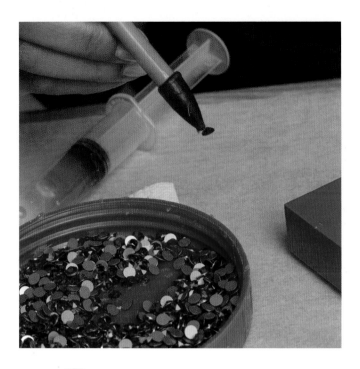
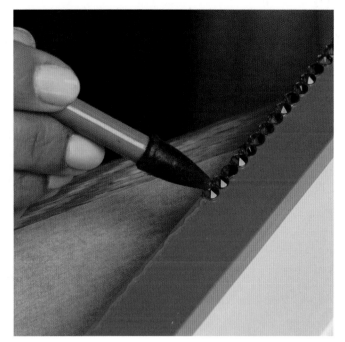

3 Using the bling tool, pick up a crystal (facet side up) and place down onto the glue. Add another stone to the glue line so that it interlocks with the first stone. Keep repeating the procedure one stone at a time.

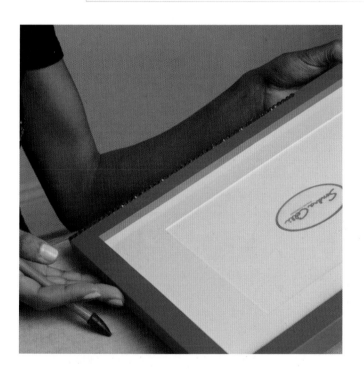
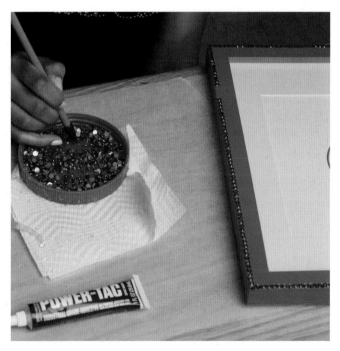

4 You want to create one long, continuous line of interlocked stones along the entire outer edge of the frame.

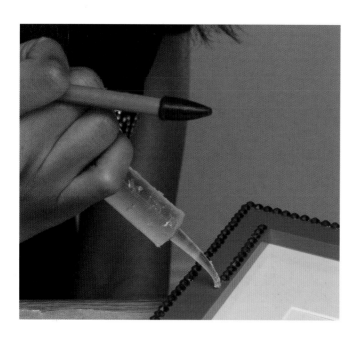
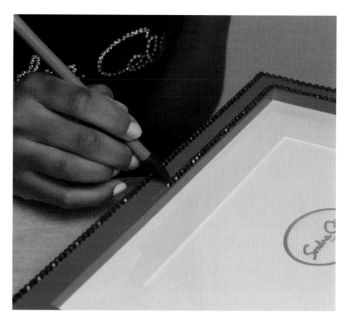

5

Once the frame has been completely outlined with stones, start lining the interior edge of the frame.

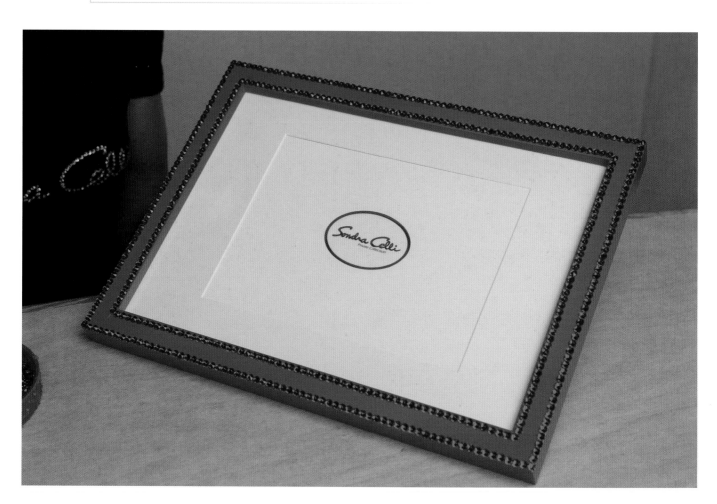

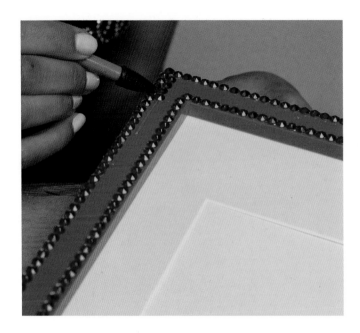
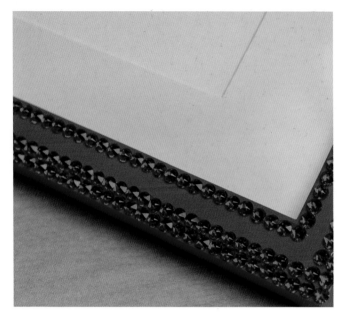

6 With both outer and inner edges trimmed, it's time to fill in the entire frame. Start by adding a row of interlocked stones on top of the row outlining the exterior edge of the frame. When that row is complete, add another row and another until you have the entire frame filled with stones.

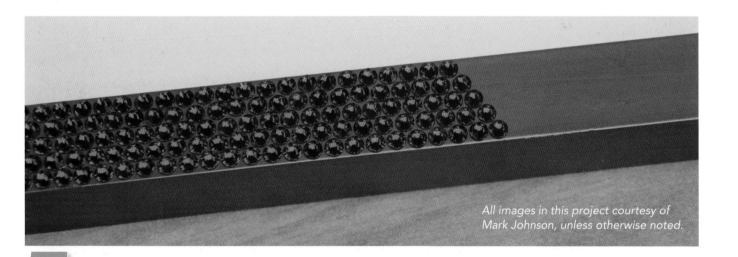

All images in this project courtesy of Mark Johnson, unless otherwise noted.

7 It took five rows of interlocked stones to fill in our frame. The number of rows will vary based on the size of frame you choose to bling.

With the Interlock technique under your belt, you are now an official Bling-ette in training!

8 Allow frame to dry completely overnight.

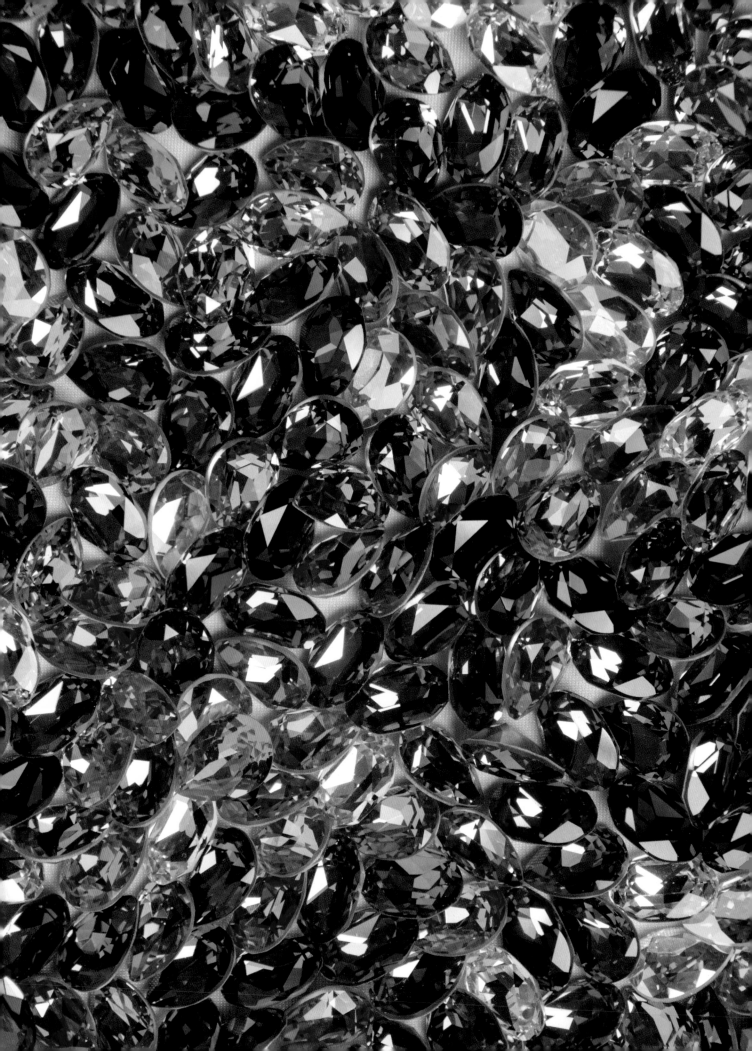

10.
Pack-and-Fade Technique

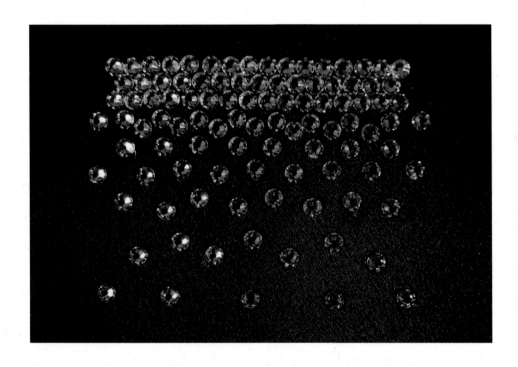

The Pack-and-Fade, also known as the "waterfall" pattern, is one of my favorite techniques. Stones are tightly packed together as with the Interlock technique, but then you begin to gradually space them farther and farther apart so that they appear to "fade" away. The Pack-and-Fade is a good way to save time and money because you don't use as many stones as you would with the Interlock, which completely packs a design.

Example of the Pack-and-Fade technique.

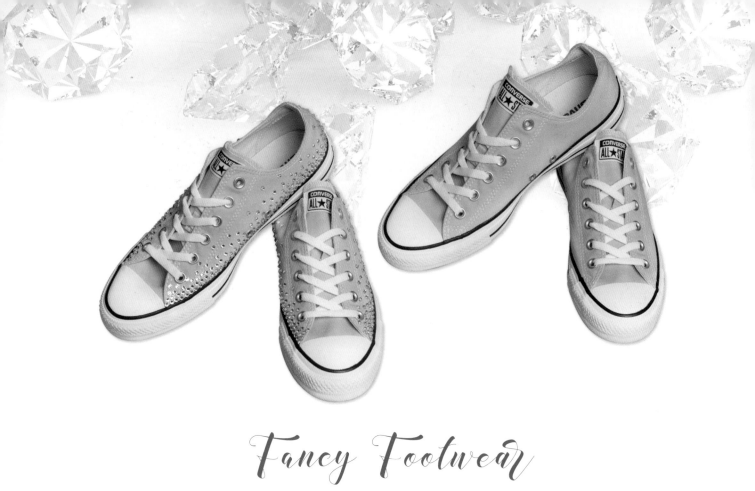

Fancy Footwear

These days it's easy to find all kinds of footwear embellished with bling: sandals, sneakers, boots, heels, even baby booties. Since they are such a popular accessory, we will use a pair of sneakers to illustrate the Pack-and-Fade technique. Refer to the Pack-and-Fade example photo above to help guide you with stone placement as you work.

Review the list of "Materials You Will Need" and the "Getting Started" guidelines in chapter 7 (page 103) before beginning any project.

1 Place a few tiny glue dots along the canvas edge of the sneaker, above the rubber trim. Leave a bit of space between each stone about half the diameter of the stone you are using. For our example we used 16ss.

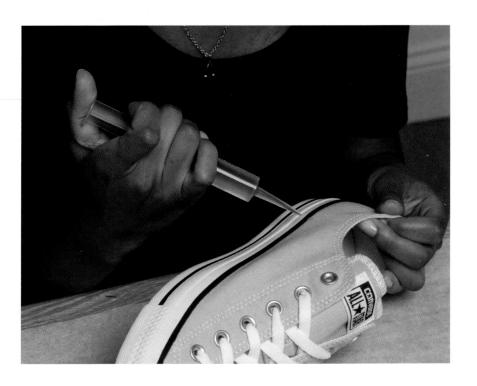

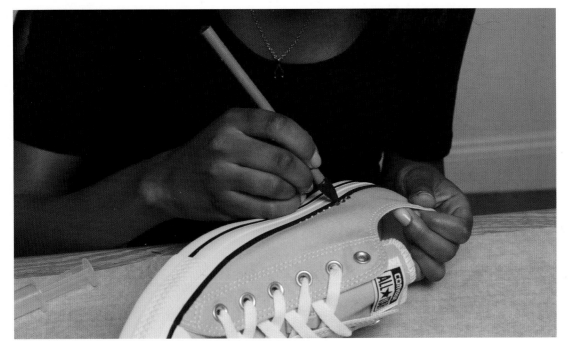

2
Using the bling tool, pick up crystals one by one and gently press down each stone onto a glue dot.

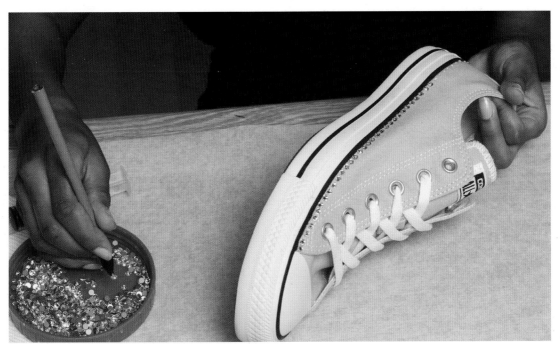

3
Continue gluing stones around the edge, stopping at the rubber toe. Leave the entire toe tip free of stones.

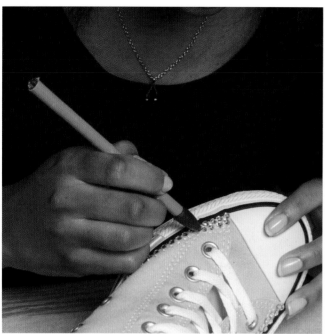 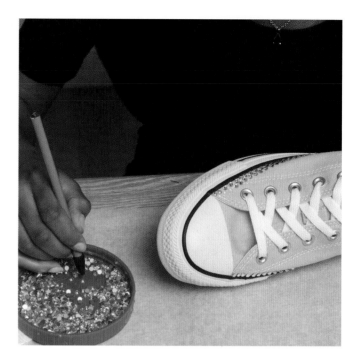

4 Once you finish the first line, begin a second row on top of the first, with the same spacing. However, when you place the second-row stones, try to center them in between two of the stones in the first row (see stone placement in Pack-and-Fade example photo above). Continue gluing stones around the sneaker in the same manner, stopping at the rubber toe. We are adding bling only to the canvas part of the sneaker.

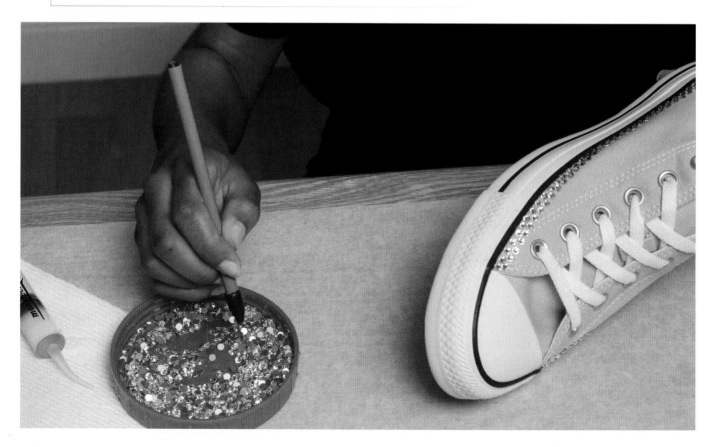

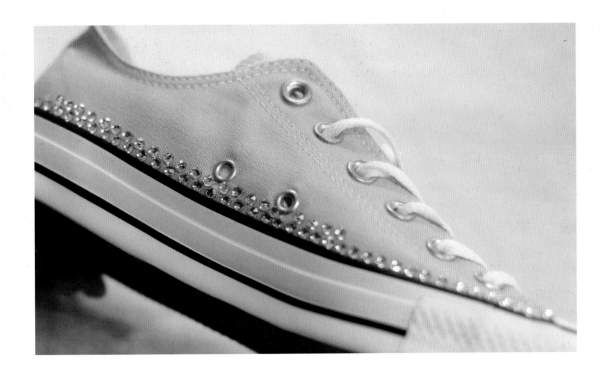

5 Create a third row of stones, spacing crystals farther apart than on the first two completed rows. Work the third row around the sneaker.

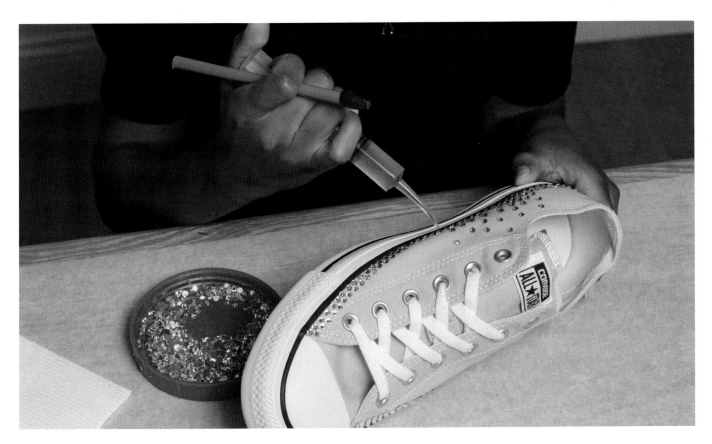

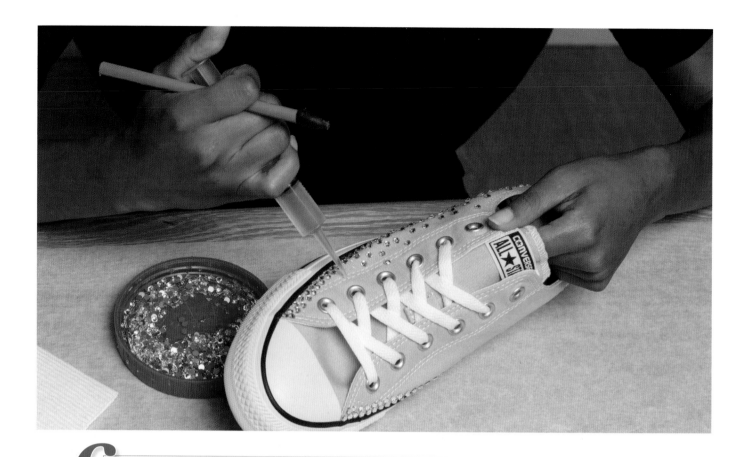

6 For rows 4 and up, begin "fading" the stones by gluing them with more and more space in between. This gives the illusion that the stones are fading away.

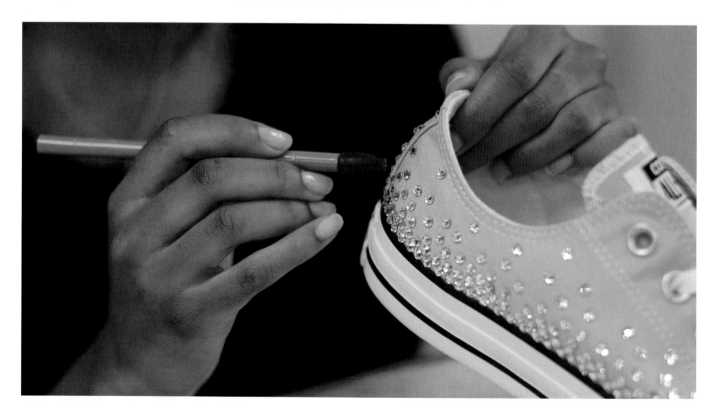

7 Add stones only up to the lace holes of the sneaker.

8 Allow sneakers to dry completely overnight.

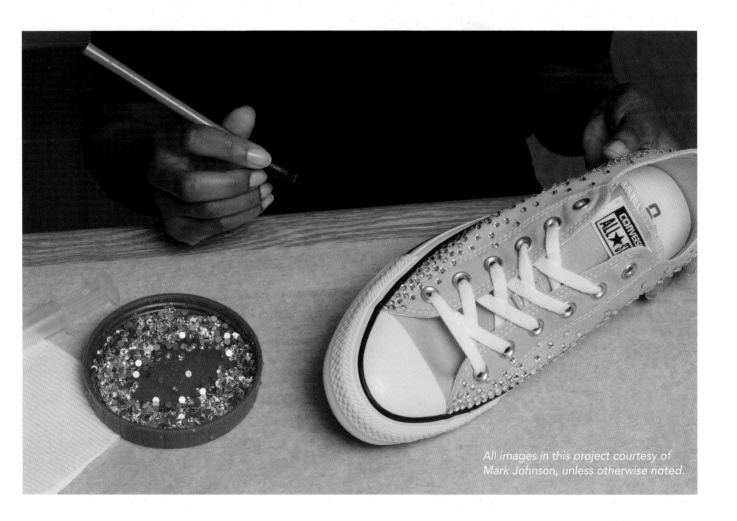

All images in this project courtesy of Mark Johnson, unless otherwise noted.

The finished Pack-and-Fade looks great. Now, that's some fancy footwork!

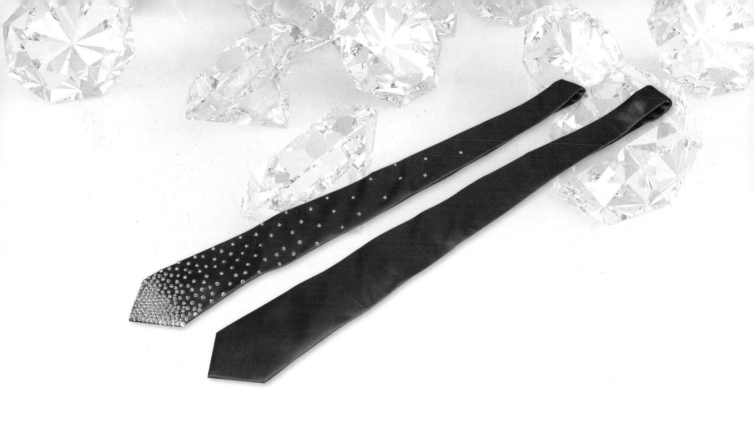

Transformed Tie

A tie tastefully accented with stones is a fun addition to any man's wardrobe. Bring out the bling for a holiday party, black-tie affair, or wedding.

Review the list of "Materials You Will Need" and the "Getting Started" guidelines in chapter 7 (page 103) before beginning any project.

1 Start by outlining the bottom tip of the tie with a row of stones tightly packed together.

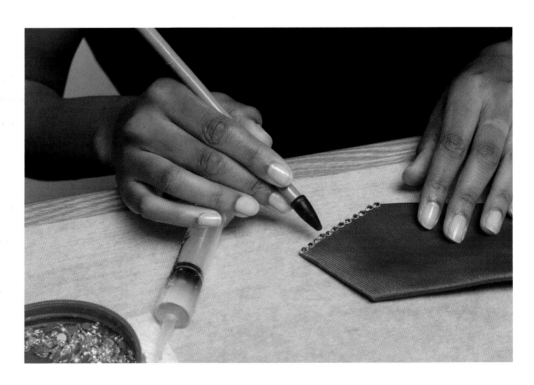

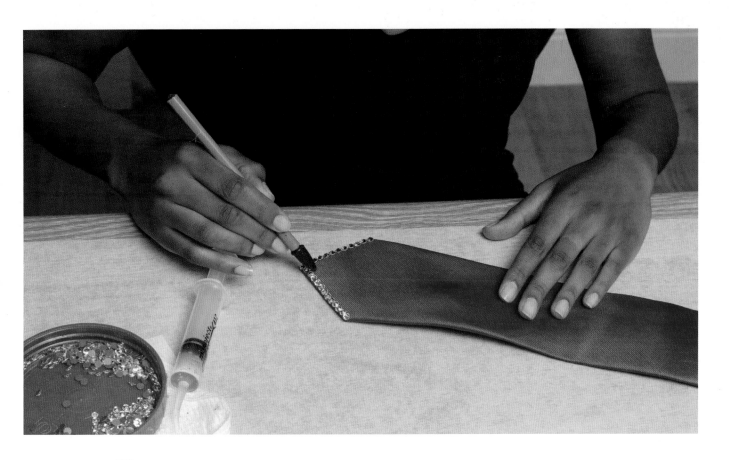

2 Now fill in the entire tip of the tie with tightly packed stones. The finished area will resemble an inverted bling triangle. This is the "Pack" part of the Pack-and-Fade. Now let's move on to the "Fade" part of the technique.

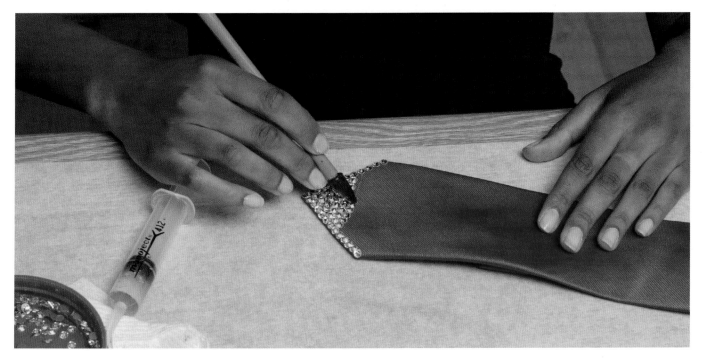

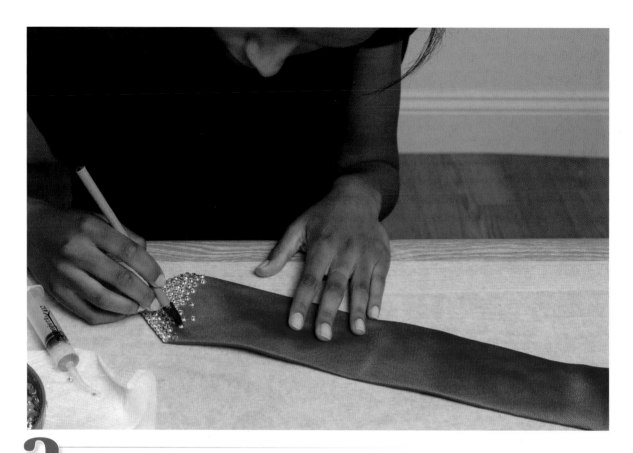

3 Begin "fading" your stones by placing them randomly and leaving more and more space in between as you work your way up the tie. Keep in mind that you want to leave about 9 to 10 inches from the top end of the tie free of stones.

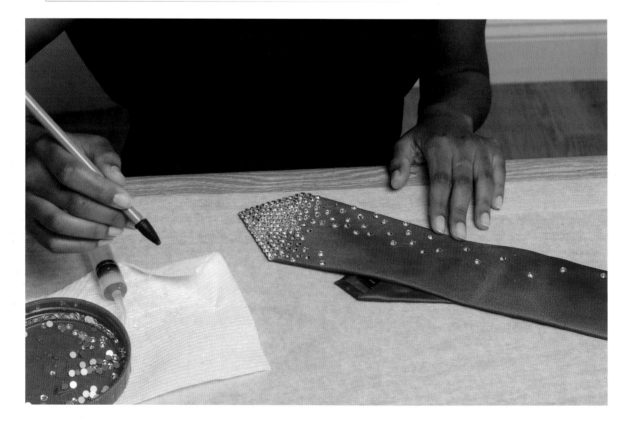

4 Allow tie to dry completely overnight. Your finished project is sure to impress and will leave people tongue-tied!

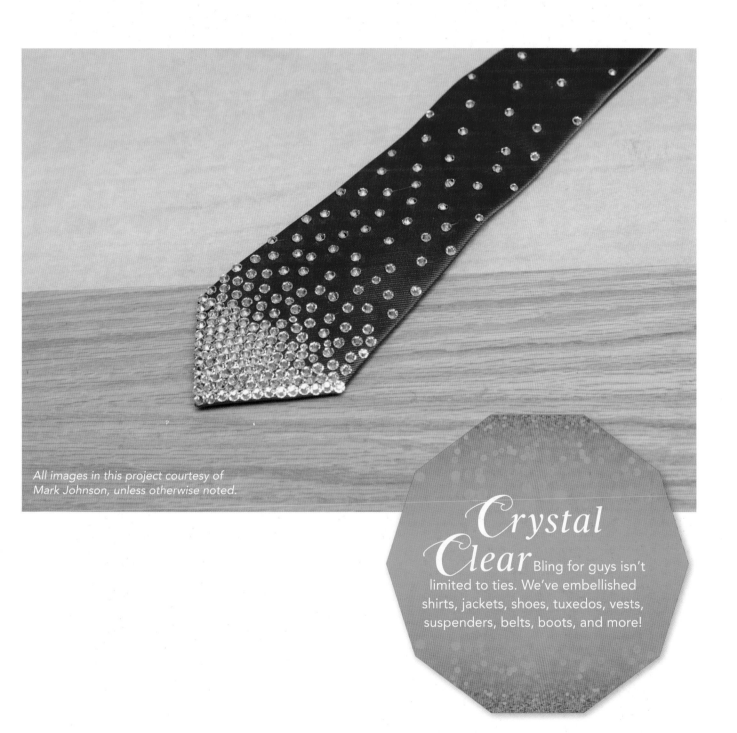

All images in this project courtesy of Mark Johnson, unless otherwise noted.

Crystal Clear Bling for guys isn't limited to ties. We've embellished shirts, jackets, shoes, tuxedos, vests, suspenders, belts, boots, and more!

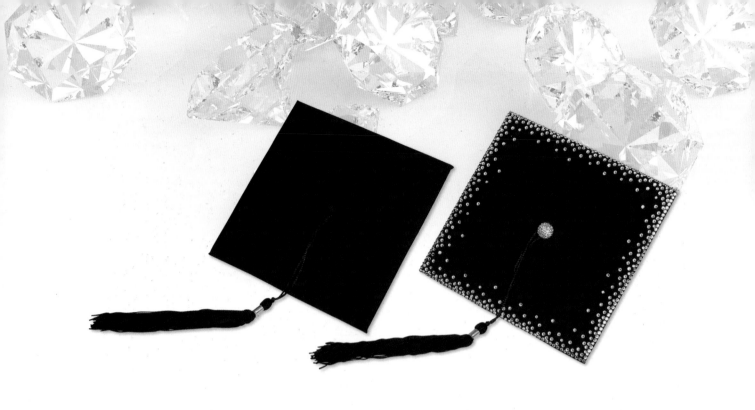

Embellished Cap

Any graduation is a momentous occasion, and one way to celebrate is by expressing your sparkling personality with an embellished graduation cap.

Review the list of "Materials You Will Need" and the "Getting Started" guidelines in chapter 7 (page 103) before beginning any project.

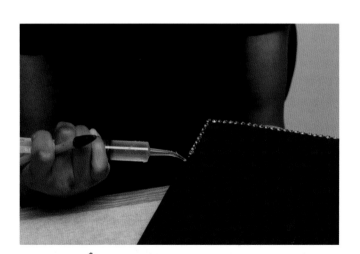

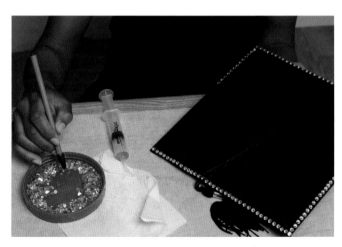

1 We are going to start embellishing the graduation cap by outlining the outer edge of the cap with a row of stones. You always want to outline a project first before filling it in with crystals. To do this, make a few glue dots on the edge and, with the bling tool, pick up a crystal (faceted side up) and gently push the stone onto the glue dot. Continue in the same manner until the entire cap has been outlined.

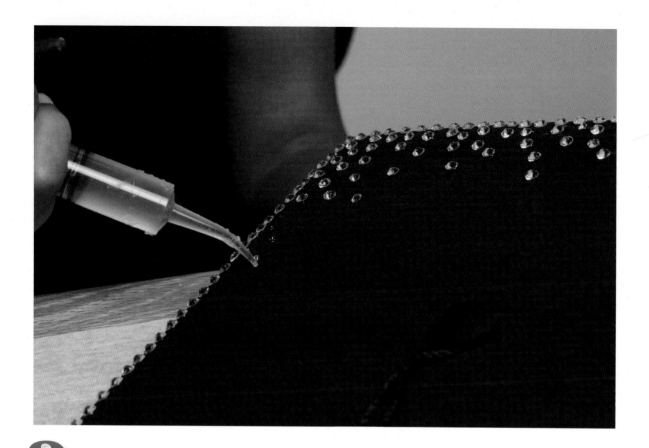

2 Just above your outline, begin to add stones randomly and with more space in between each stone. Work your way slightly inward toward the center of the cap as you go. Complete all four sides of the cap.

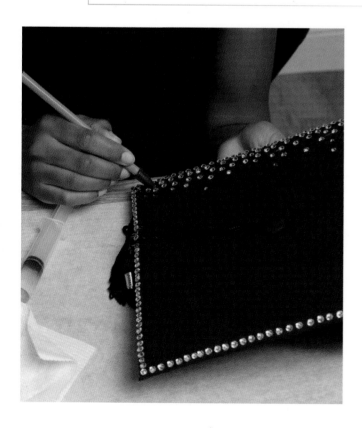

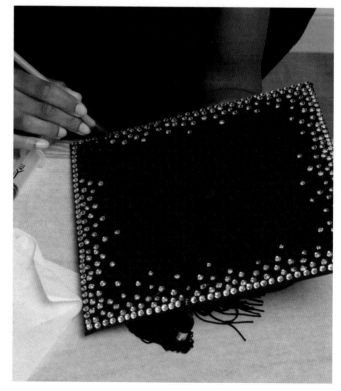

3

Finish off the cap by tightly packing the button in the center with crystals.

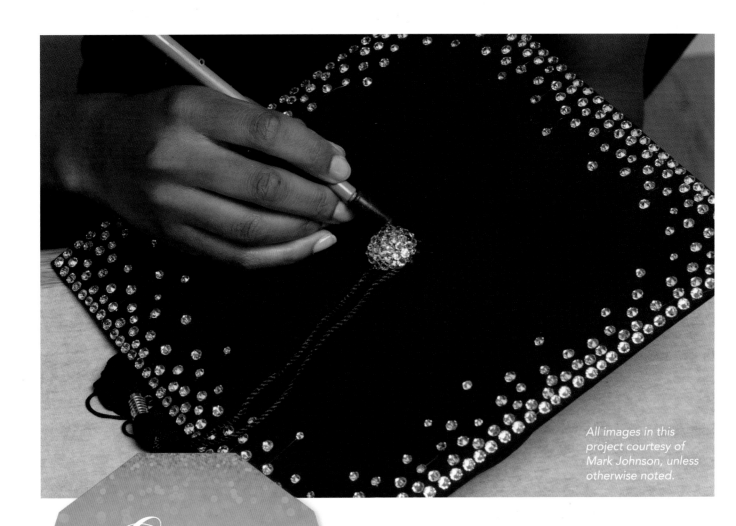

All images in this project courtesy of Mark Johnson, unless otherwise noted.

Crystal Clear

The Pack-and-Fade technique is also used to create the ombré effect, when you mix different shades of stones together that are packed and faded from dark to light (or vice versa). You will learn about that technique in the next chapter.

4

Allow cap to dry completely overnight. Hats off to you for your terrific topper!

11.
Crystal Waterfall (Ombré) Technique

Crystal Waterfall is the term I use to describe this next technique because the pattern resembles a waterfall, with stones starting tightly packed together in a wave and then gradually cascading away. However, the technique is better known as ombré, a French word used to describe the striking effect you get when different shades of a color gradually fade into one other. The fade can progress from lighter to darker tones or vice versa. To get the best effect with ombré requires a minimum of three different shades.

The ombré technique actually combines two techniques we learned in earlier chapters: the Interlock and the Pack-and-Fade.

Crystal Clear
Swarovski® offers an overwhelming range of color stones to choose from. Your biggest hurdle will be deciding which complementary shades you like best for your ombré projects. Purchase a small supply of stones so you can see firsthand how well they blend together before buying the entire inventory you need to get started.

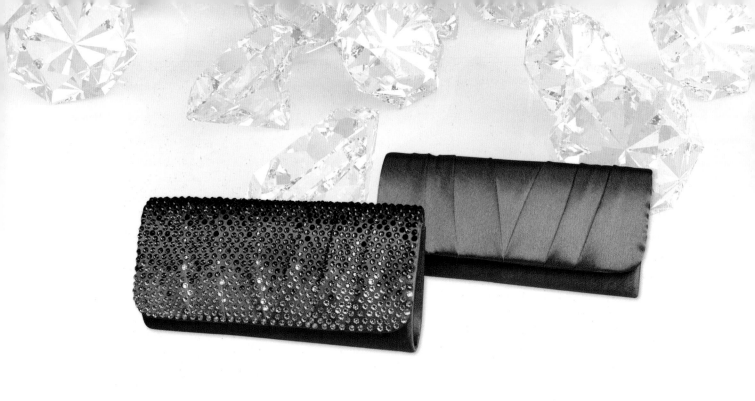

Crystal Clutch

Forget the bubbly and add some sparkling effervescence to an evening out with a crystal clutch! Review the list of "Materials You Will Need" and the "Getting Started" guidelines in chapter 7 (page 103) before beginning any project.

1

Using T-pins (or straight pins), mark where you want the transitions from one tone into another to begin. The pins will be your guide as you work. Since we will use three tones in our example, we have divided the clutch into thirds. Our ombré graduates from dark into light by starting with Jet crystals and then fading into two lighter tones: Black Diamond, then Clear.

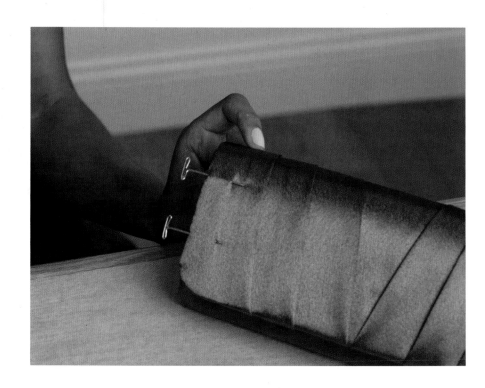

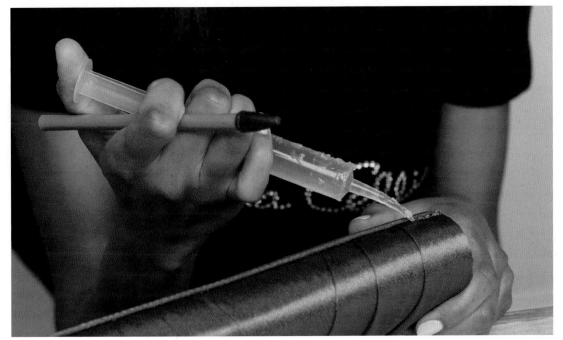

2 Start at the top of the clutch by applying a short, thin line of glue and then placing Jet stones on the line side by side in a tight row.

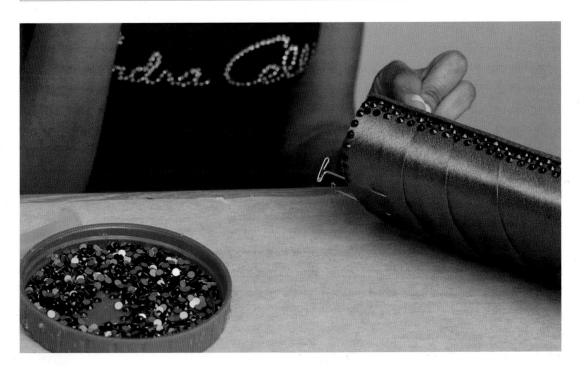

3 Once you have completed the entire top row, create a second line of stones directly underneath.

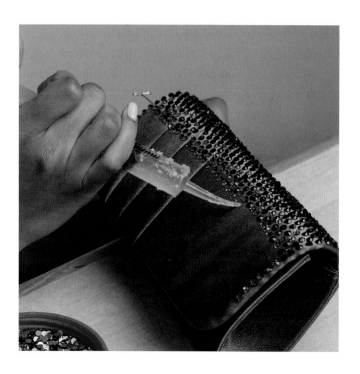
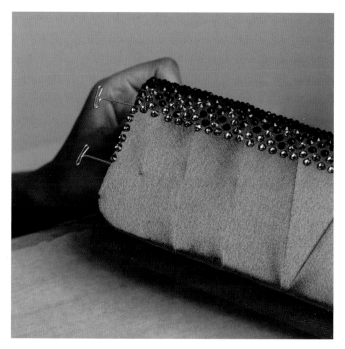

4 Continue making rows in this manner until you come to your first pin marker. This is where you will begin adding a few stones of your second color into the row at random (in our case, Black Diamond).

5 With each new additional row, place more of the second-color stones, working to fade out the first color (in our case, Jet stones) completely. You should be at or very near to the second pin marker when you reach this point.

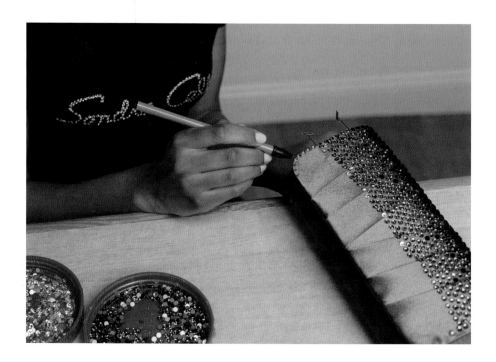

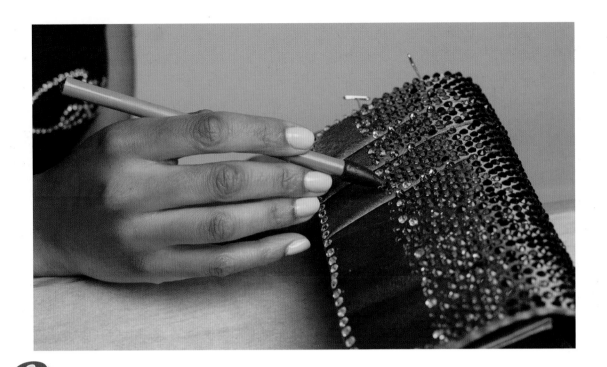

6

At the second pin, start to randomly introduce your third, and final, color (in our case, Clear). Again, begin sprinkling Clear stones into the rows until you have completely phased out Jet, and finish using only Black Diamond. After you have entirely eliminated the Black Diamond stones from the rows, continue to the end with just Clear stones.

7

Allow clutch to dry completely overnight.

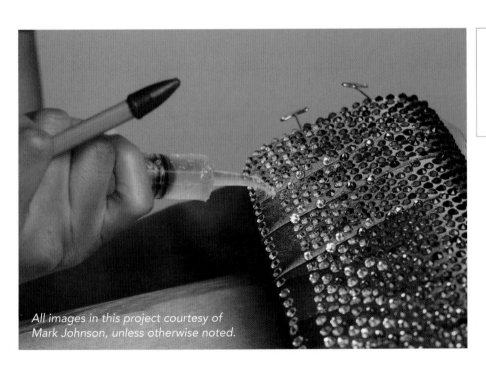

All images in this project courtesy of Mark Johnson, unless otherwise noted.

The finished clutch makes for a striking accessory.

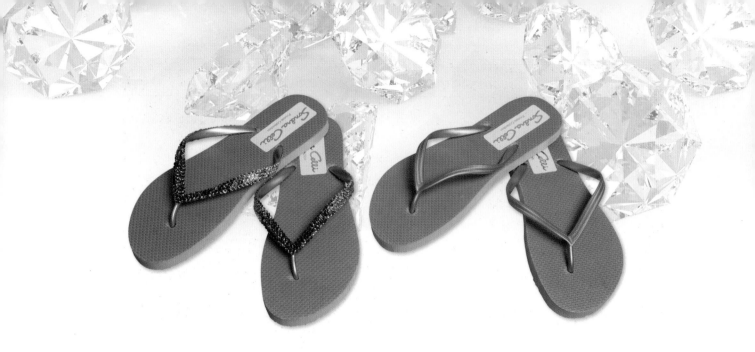

Fab Flops

Add some razzle dazzle to your summer with a bit of beach bling!

Review the list of "Materials You Will Need" and the "Getting Started" guidelines in chapter 7 (page 103) before beginning any project.

1

Divide the flip-flops into thirds by making a small mark using a gel pen. This will be the guide to show you where you want to begin and end each of the three color tones you will be using for your Ombré. For our example we will transition from dark to light, using stones in colors of Fern, Peridot, and Crystal.

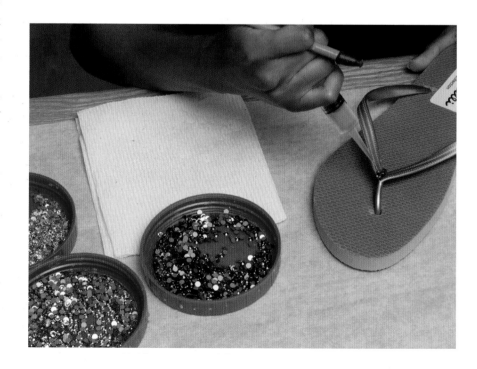

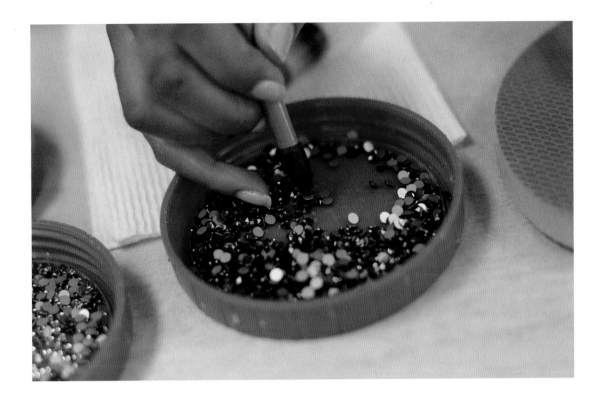

2 Begin the Ombré motif at the top of the flip-flop, near the toe strap. Start with your first stone color (we used Fern). Make a few glue dots, pick up stones with the bling tool, and gently press stones onto the dots. Pack stones tightly together as you glue them onto the flip-flops. For our example, size 16ss stones were used.

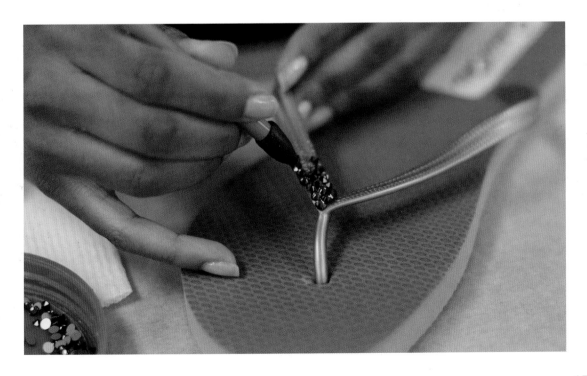

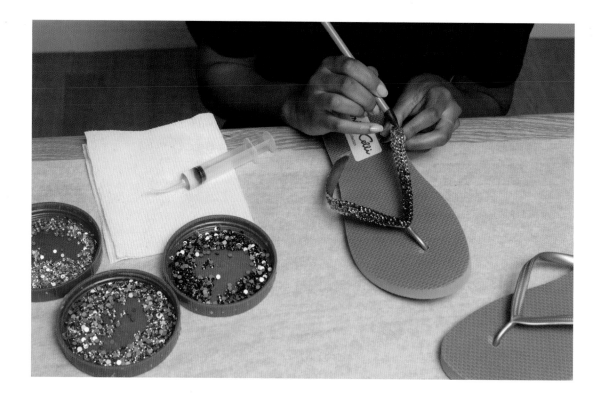

3

Begin to introduce your second color (we used Peridot) by randomly sprinkling in a few stones among the darker Fern stones. Continue adding more of the second-color crystals while gradually fading out the first-color crystals until the first color has completely disappeared and you are using only your second color. This should happen about one-third of the way down the straps.

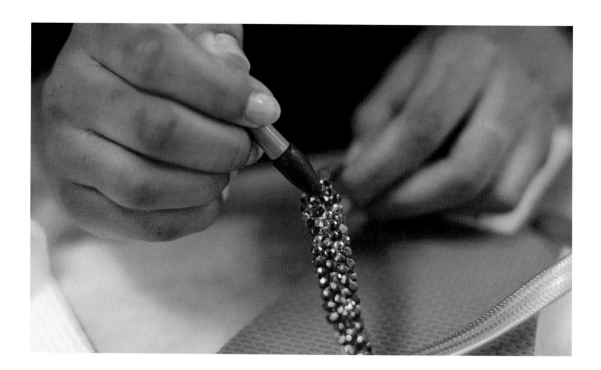

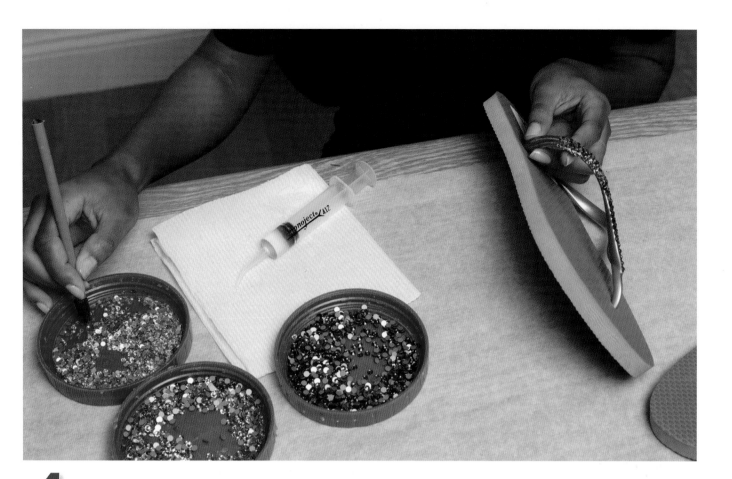

4

About two-thirds of the way down, randomly introduce your third and final stone color (we used Crystal). Continue adding more and more Crystal stones while using fewer and fewer Peridot until the Peridot has completely disappeared and you are using only Crystal.

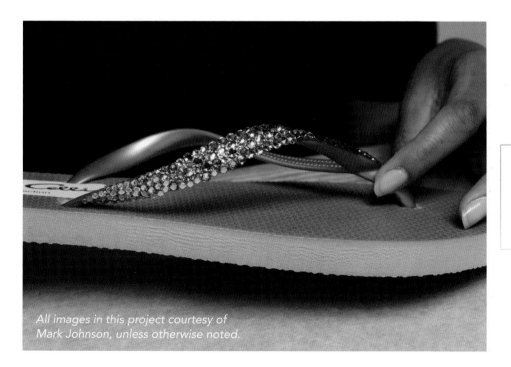

All images in this project courtesy of Mark Johnson, unless otherwise noted.

5

Allow flip-flops to dry completely overnight.

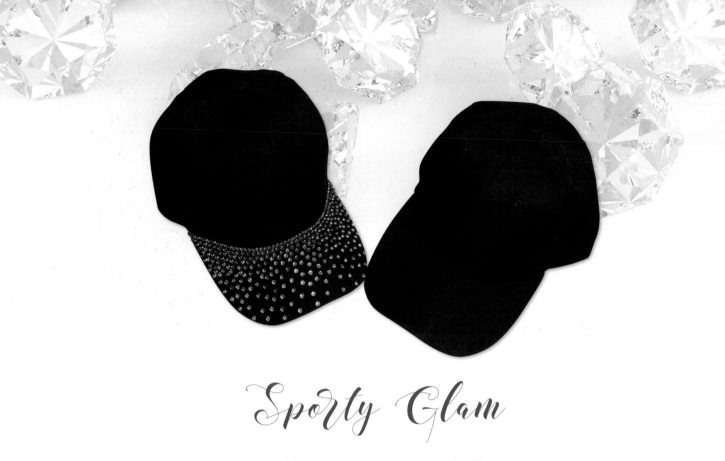

Sporty Glam

For this next project we'll accent the bill of a baseball hat with crystals in a loose Ombré pattern using Fuchsia, Rose, and Light Rose stones. We start using only Fuchsia stones tightly packed together in rows. As we progress toward the outer edge of the visor, we randomly add in our second color while fading out and eventually eliminating stones of the first color. Find a point at which to add the third color while fading out the second color entirely. You will end up creating the final few rows by using only Light Rose.

Again, as you fade colors in and out, you'll also be widening the stones' placement, leaving more and more space between crystals.

Review the list of "Materials You Will Need" and the "Getting Started" guidelines in chapter 7 (page 103) before beginning any project.

Above It's time to switch it up! Give that boring baseball hat a bit of glam and you'll knock it out of the park!

1

Start your Ombré motif where the visor meets at the bottom seam of the hat crown. Apply a narrow line of adhesive.

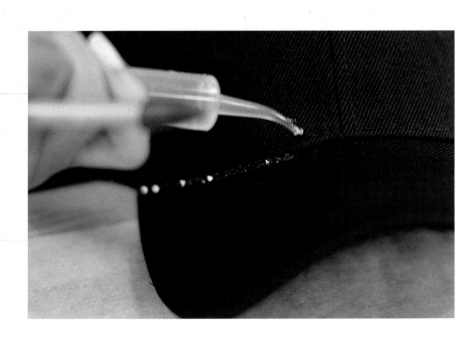

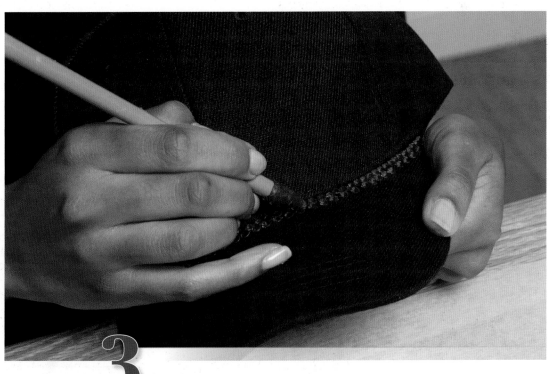

2 Using your bling tool, press stones down onto the glue in a tight row along the visor seam. This is row 1.

3 Create a row 2 directly above row 1, but begin to leave a bit of space in between the stones in the row. Add row 3 above row 2 and leave slightly more space in between the stones.

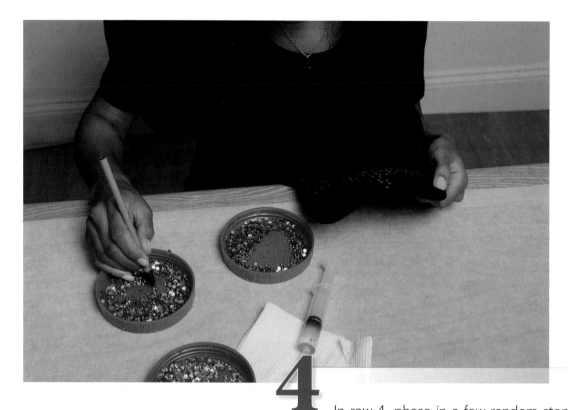

4 In row 4, phase in a few random stones of your second color into the row. As you work, you want to add more of the second color while beginning to phase out the first color until it completely disappears.

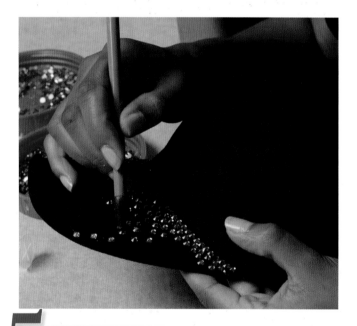

5 From row 5 up to the visor edge, your rows will now break up to become randomly placed stones. Add in your third and final color (in our example, Light Rose) as you move toward the edge of the hat while gradually decreasing the second color. For the last few rows, only Light Rose stones (your final color) are used.

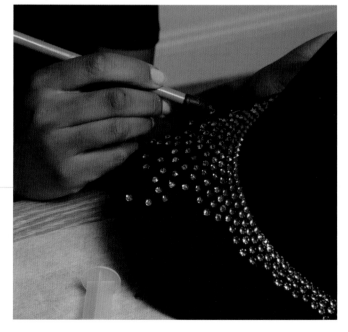

6 Allow hat to dry completely overnight.

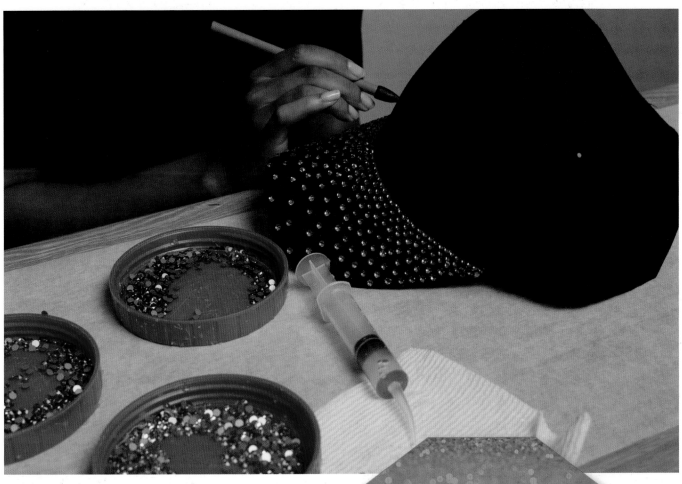

All images in this project courtesy of Mark Johnson, unless otherwise noted.

Crystal Clear

The number of rows you make and where your color transitions take place will change depending on the size of the object you are working on and where you decide that you want to introduce a new color. The Ombré technique is a rather loose and somewhat random pattern, so do not make yourself crazy trying to be exact with stone placement. The more you bling, the better you will get.

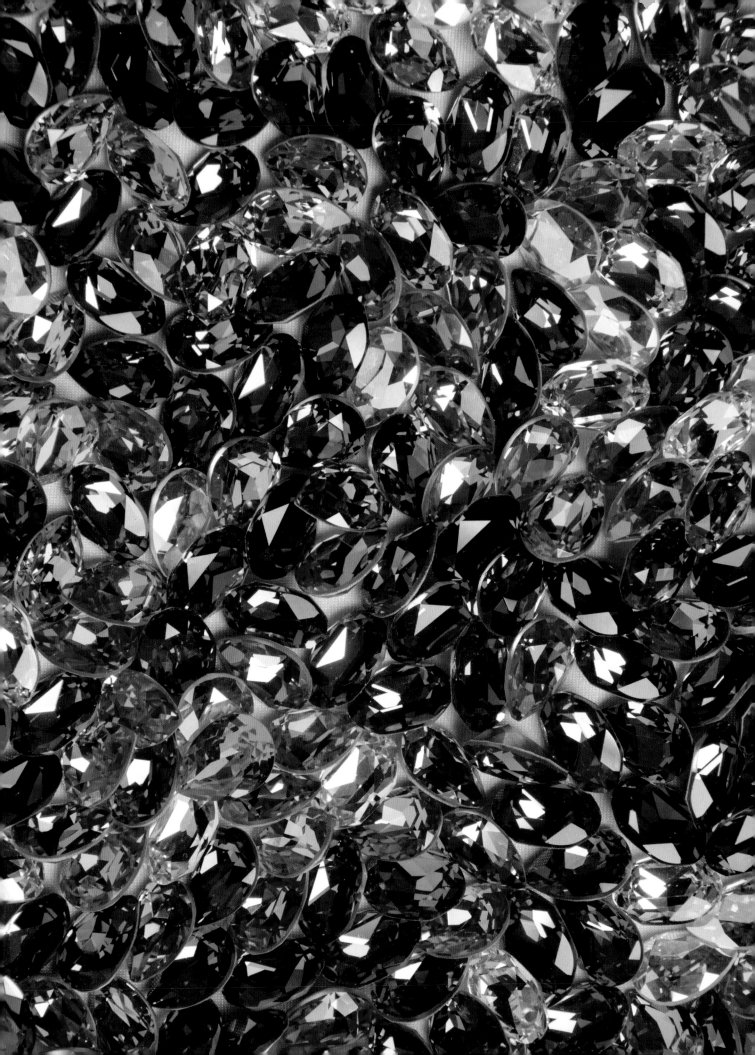

12.
Highlighting Lace

A great way to save money but make a big impact is to highlight lace fabric with crystals. You do not need a lot of stones, because the pattern in the lace already entertains the eyes, yet when you accent the lace with a little bling you can transform it into something extraordinary.

Review the list of "Materials You Will Need" and the "Getting Started" guidelines in chapter 7 (page 103) before beginning any project.

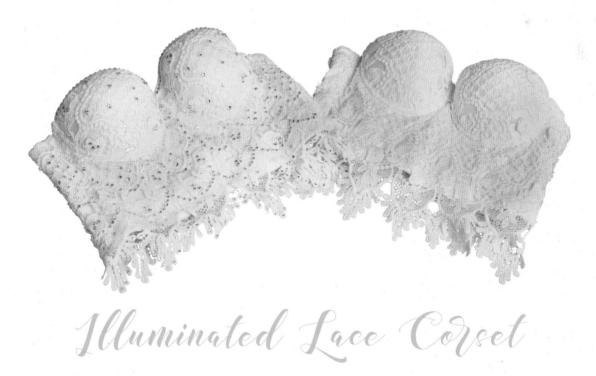

Illuminated Lace Corset

Highlighting lace with sparkling crystals is more of a free-style technique. There is no design formula to follow, making it very easy. The object is to adapt the stone placement to the lace's pattern.

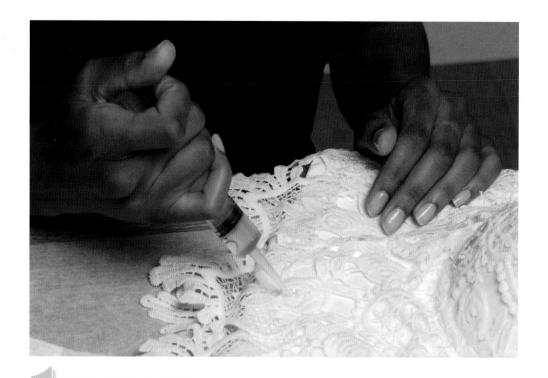

1 Start by putting a few glue dots on random areas of the lace.

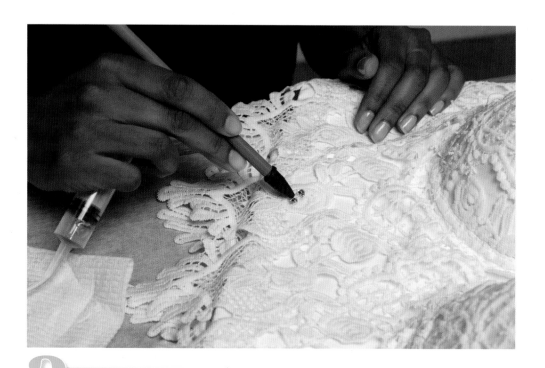

2 Using the bling tool, pick up crystals (faceted side up) and gently press stones into the dots on the lace fabric.

3 Continue adding stones, taking time to stop every so often to review their placement. You want to avoid bunching too-many stones close together or leaving wide-open areas blank.

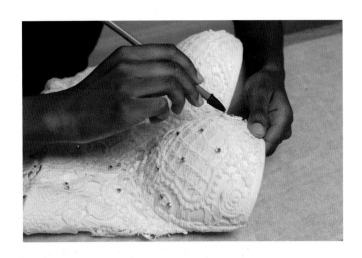

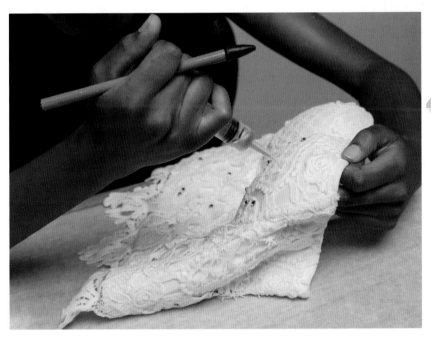

4 For a different flair, you can locate a pattern within the lace and highlight it with stones.

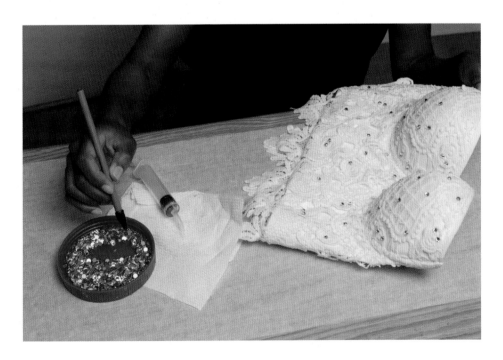

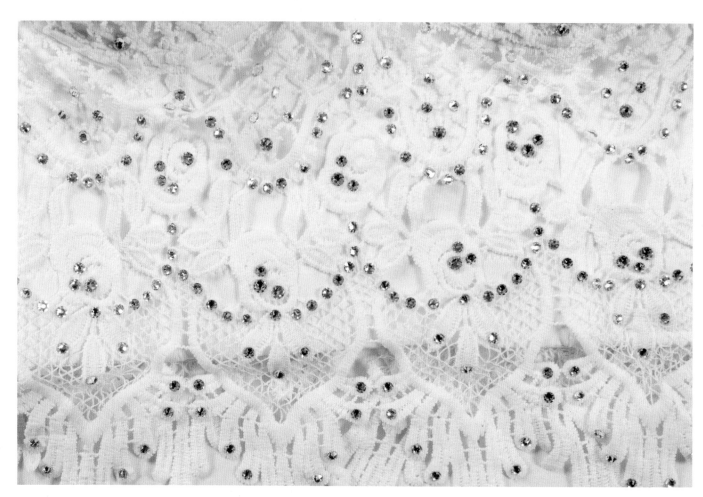

*All images in this project courtesy of
Mark Johnson, unless otherwise noted.*

5 Allow the corset to dry completely overnight.

*Mix it up, be spontaneous, and
have fun as you highlight.
The outcome is phenomenal!*

13.
Swirls and Florals

Two popular bling patterns are my whirling swirls and flourishing florals. Both patterns add interest and movement to a design. Over the years I have used them on dresses, shoes, and even accent pillows.

Both patterns are included in this book for you to use. (See detailed instructions in the next two projects.)

Tee-rrific!

Review the list of "Materials You Will Need" and the "Getting Started" guidelines in chapter 7 (page 103) before beginning any project. In addition, you will need a pair of scissors and a piece of cardboard to insert inside the T-shirt to hold the fabric flat. The cardboard should be large enough to cover the area you are going to stone.

Finally, if the fabric of the T-shirt you select is excessively thin or sheer, place parchment paper in between the shirt and cardboard. Otherwise the T-shirt could end up sticking to the cardboard when you glue stones on the shirt.

Add a little bling flourish to a tired tee.
Courtesy of Mark Johnson

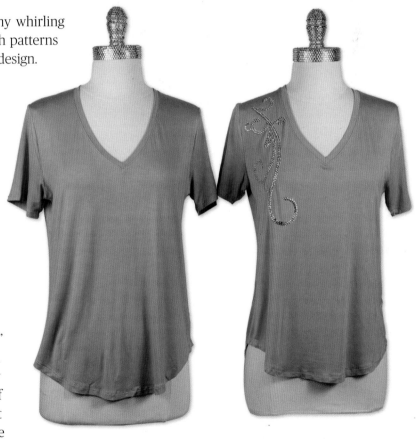

1 Select the color and style of T-shirt you want, then wash and dry it. You want to ensure that any shrinkage of the fabric happens before adding the stones.

2

Iron out any wrinkles so the T-shirt will lie flat. This makes it easier to apply the crystals.

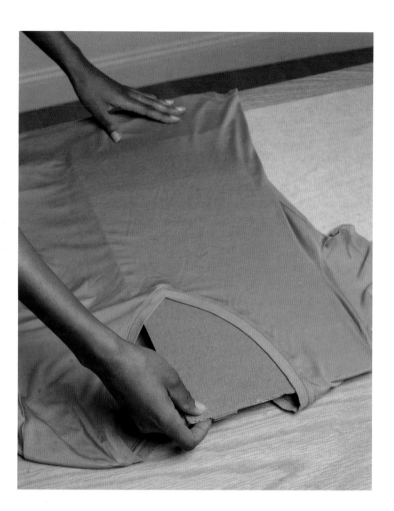

3

Insert a sheet of cardboard inside the T-shirt to ensure that the shirt lies flat. Do not overstretch it.

4

Using a pair of scissors, cut out the Swirls stencil (page 169).

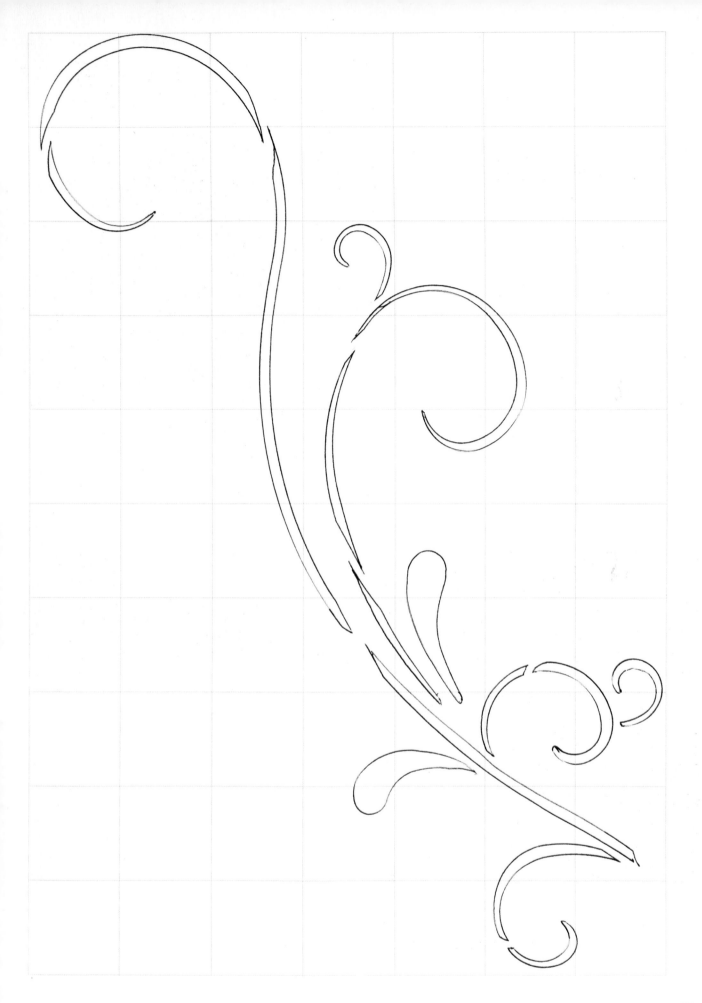

Swirls pattern stencil.

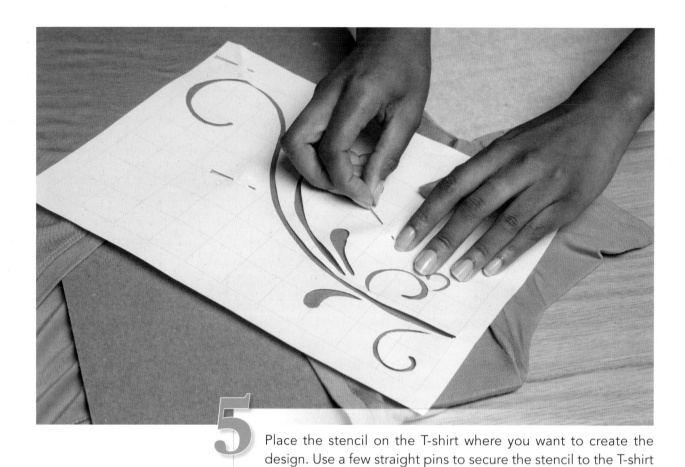

5 Place the stencil on the T-shirt where you want to create the design. Use a few straight pins to secure the stencil to the T-shirt so it won't move around as you trace.

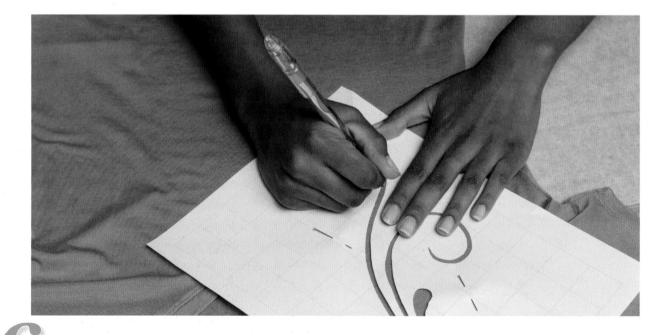

6 Lightly trace the swirls onto the T-shirt using a gel pen. Then unpin and remove the stencil. (For our sample we placed the pattern so that the swirls would adorn only one side of the T-shirt. You can bling both sides if you prefer; just allow the first side to dry completely before blinging the other side.)

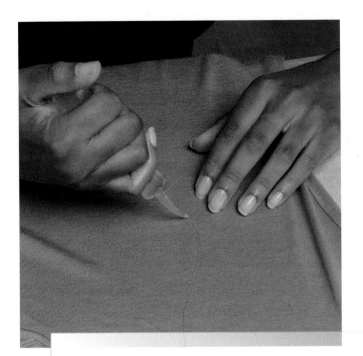
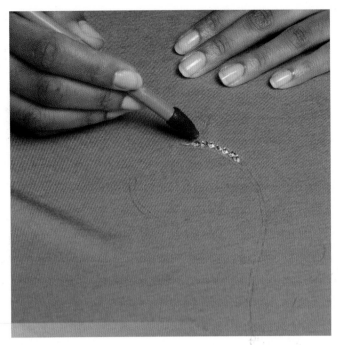

7 Select a starting point on the design and apply a narrow line of glue, following along the gel pen tracings you drew. Work only a few inches at a time to keep it manageable. Use the bling tool to place the stones on the glue lines in a tight row. Continue working in this manner, only a few inches at a time.

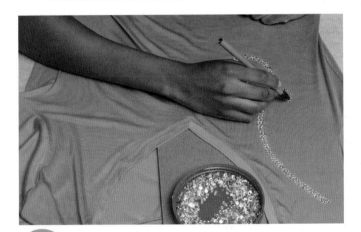

8 When you have completed a row of stones, go back and add your second row, interlocked to the first. Move on to another part of the motif until you have blinged out the entire pattern. Allow the T-shirt to completely dry overnight on the cardboard.

9

Note: Always hand-wash your blinged-out tee using mild detergent and lay flat to dry.

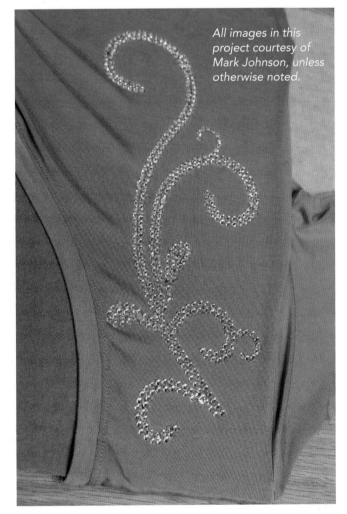

All images in this project courtesy of Mark Johnson, unless otherwise noted.

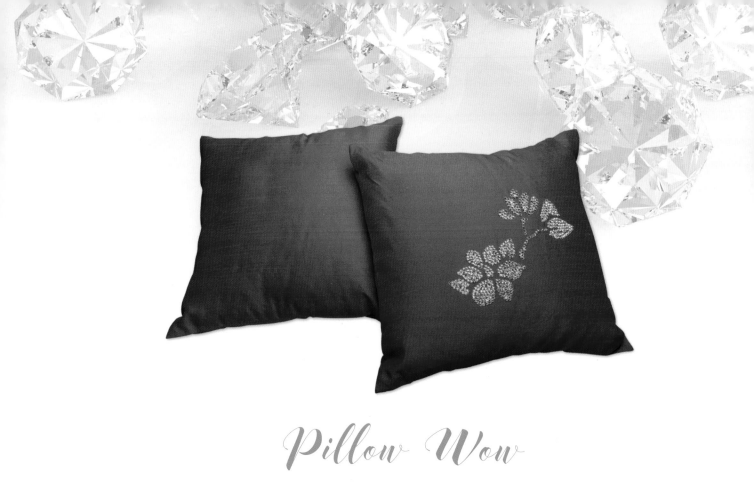

Pillow Wow

Throw pillows make great accents for almost any room in your home. So that will be our next DIY bling project using a floral flourish!

Review the list of "Materials You Will Need" and the "Getting Started" guidelines in chapter 7 (page 103) before beginning any project.

1 Choose a pillow with a plain surface in the color, size, and shape of your choice.

2 Using a pair of scissors, cut out the Florals stencil (page 173).

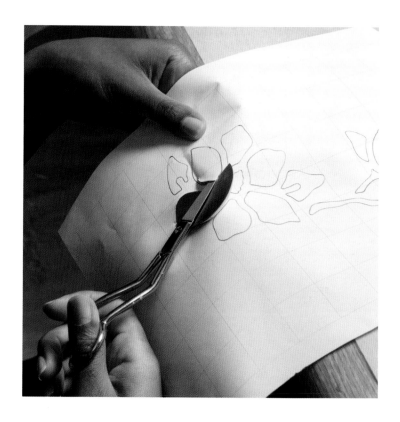

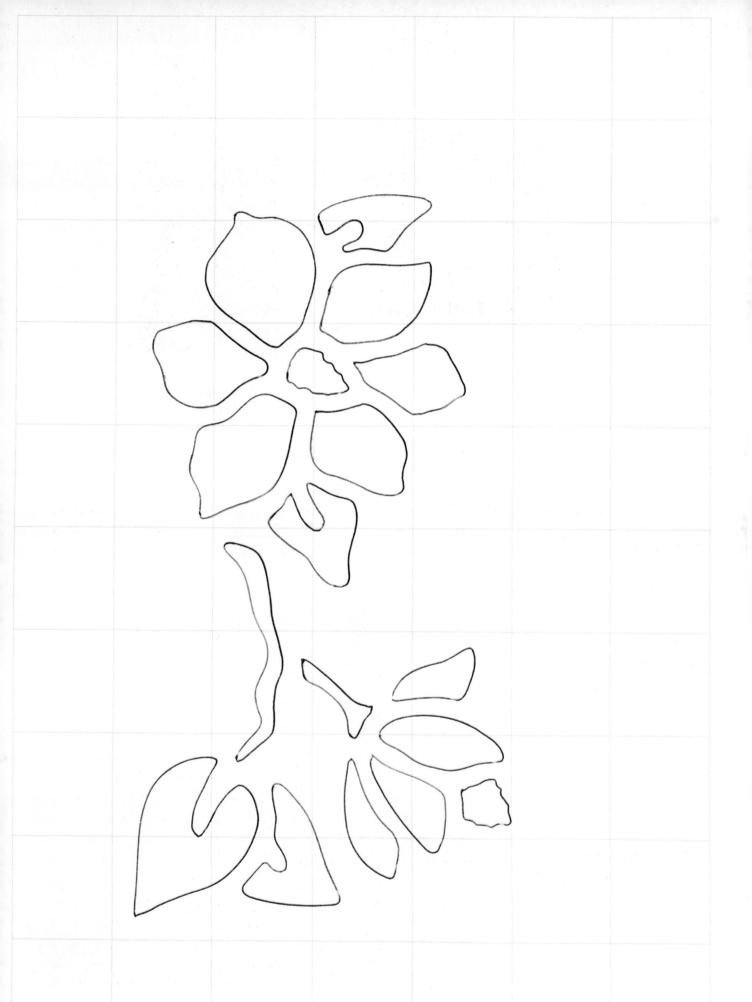

Florals pattern stencil.

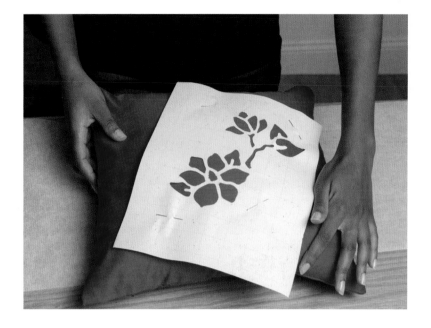

3 Pin the stencil securely to pillow using straight pins.

4 Using a gel pen, lightly trace the entire floral pattern onto the pillow fabric, then unpin and remove the stencil.

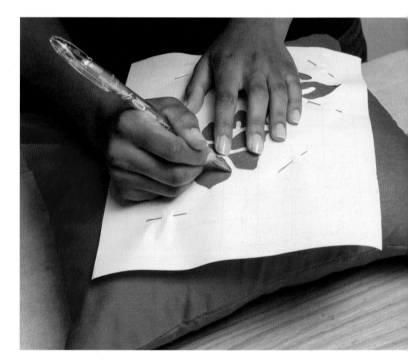

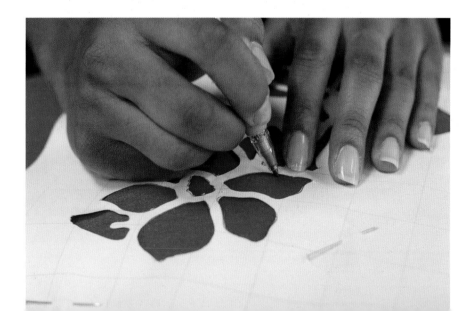

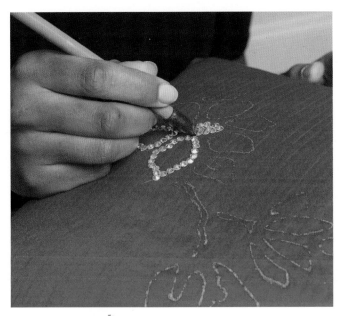
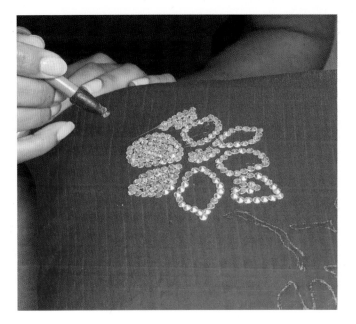

5

Begin outlining small areas of the design with glue and applying stones to those outlines. After you have completely outlined the entire design with stones, start filling in the designs with stones.

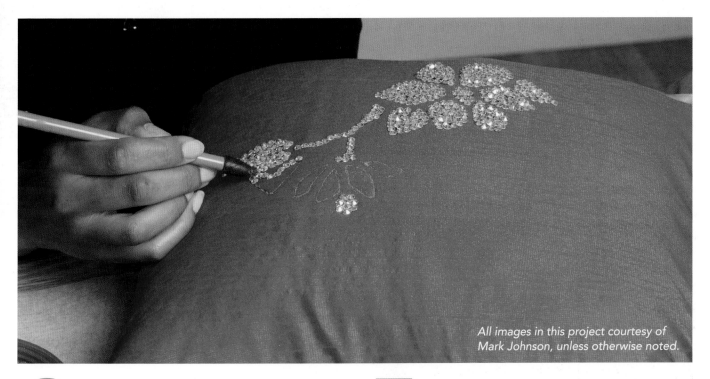

All images in this project courtesy of Mark Johnson, unless otherwise noted.

6

Fill in the entire floral pattern with stones tightly packed together.

7

Allow the pillow to completely dry overnight.

14.
The Power of Bling

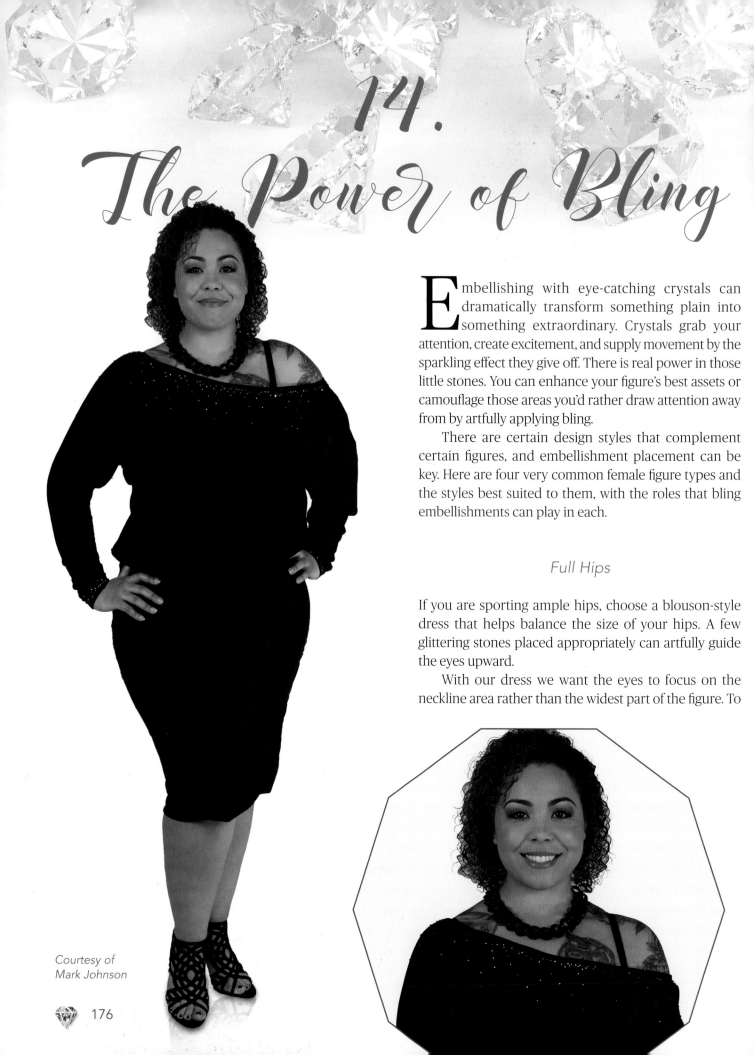

Embellishing with eye-catching crystals can dramatically transform something plain into something extraordinary. Crystals grab your attention, create excitement, and supply movement by the sparkling effect they give off. There is real power in those little stones. You can enhance your figure's best assets or camouflage those areas you'd rather draw attention away from by artfully applying bling.

There are certain design styles that complement certain figures, and embellishment placement can be key. Here are four very common female figure types and the styles best suited to them, with the roles that bling embellishments can play in each.

Full Hips

If you are sporting ample hips, choose a blouson-style dress that helps balance the size of your hips. A few glittering stones placed appropriately can artfully guide the eyes upward.

With our dress we want the eyes to focus on the neckline area rather than the widest part of the figure. To

*Courtesy of
Mark Johnson*

176

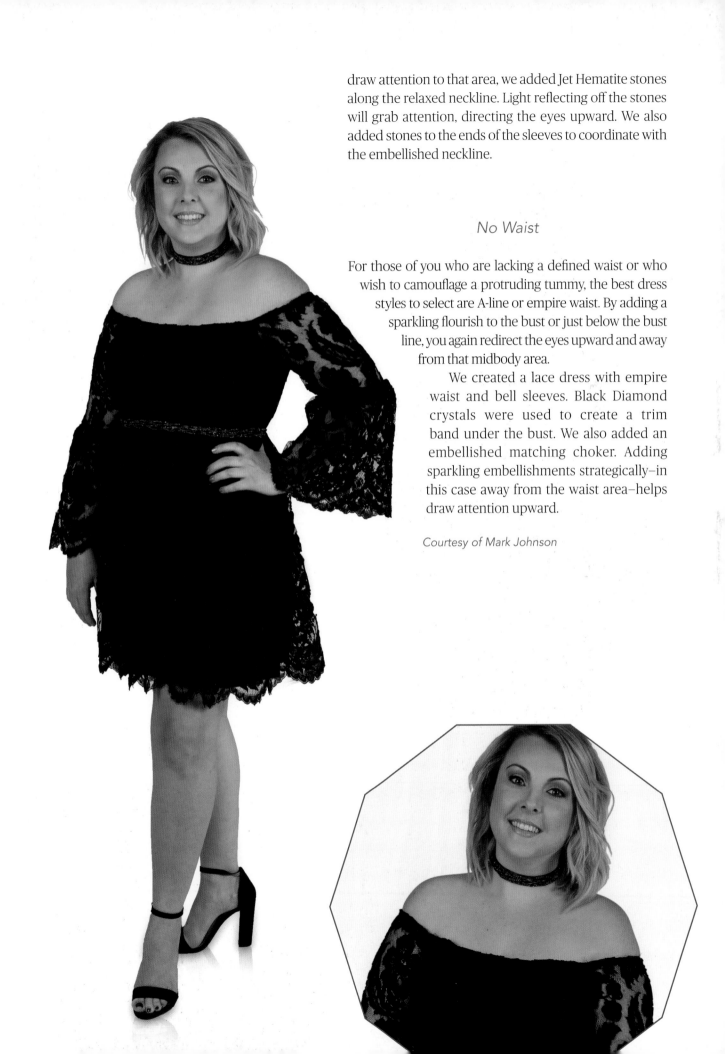

draw attention to that area, we added Jet Hematite stones along the relaxed neckline. Light reflecting off the stones will grab attention, directing the eyes upward. We also added stones to the ends of the sleeves to coordinate with the embellished neckline.

No Waist

For those of you who are lacking a defined waist or who wish to camouflage a protruding tummy, the best dress styles to select are A-line or empire waist. By adding a sparkling flourish to the bust or just below the bust line, you again redirect the eyes upward and away from that midbody area.

We created a lace dress with empire waist and bell sleeves. Black Diamond crystals were used to create a trim band under the bust. We also added an embellished matching choker. Adding sparkling embellishments strategically—in this case away from the waist area—helps draw attention upward.

Courtesy of Mark Johnson

Big Bust

To help with a big bust, first look for a high-quality bra offering substantial support. Once you have the appropriate foundation, search for a wrap-style dress that will accentuate the waist rather than the bust line. Consider the "less is more" guideline and avoid plunging necklines.

With our dress we added a large statement piece to the side of the waist, along with a burst of Jet Hematite stones spraying out in all directions, to draw the eyes downward. Stones were also used to trim the edges of the three-quarter-length sleeves.

Courtesy of Mark Johnson

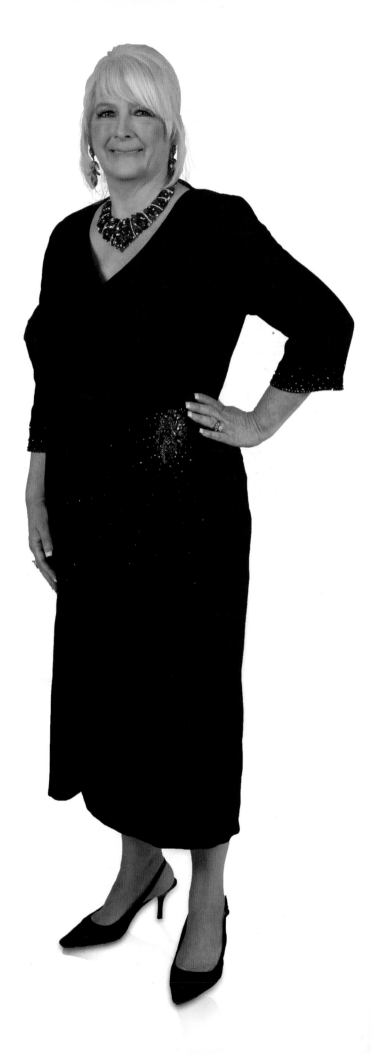

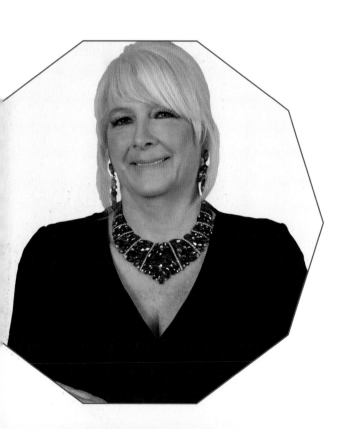

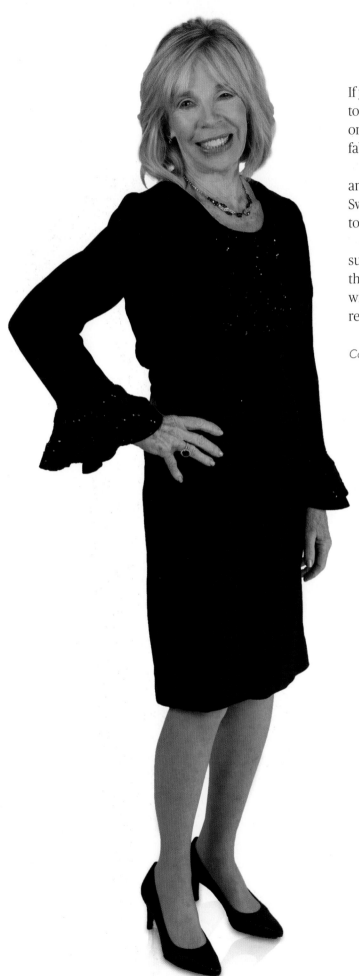

Small Bust

If you are dealing with a case of "less is less" and you want to enhance the chest area, a great way to instantly improve on a small bust is to add lace or any other dimensional fabric to the bodice. This adds fullness and interest.

For our dress we added a beautiful Alençon lace and highlighted the entire bust area with Jet Hematite Swarovski® crystals. The same crystals were also added to the bell sleeves of the short bolero jacket.

Don't be afraid to add a few sparkling accessories, such as necklaces or bracelets that coordinate, to pull the entire ensemble together. Bling plus more bling is a winning formula if done correctly. Remember, it won't really zing without the bling!

Courtesy of Mark Johnson

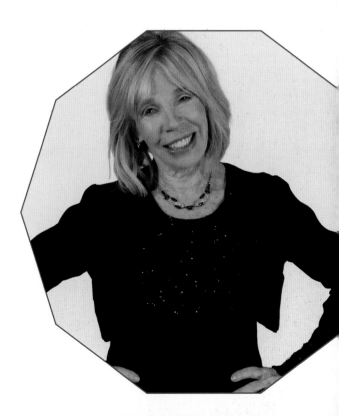

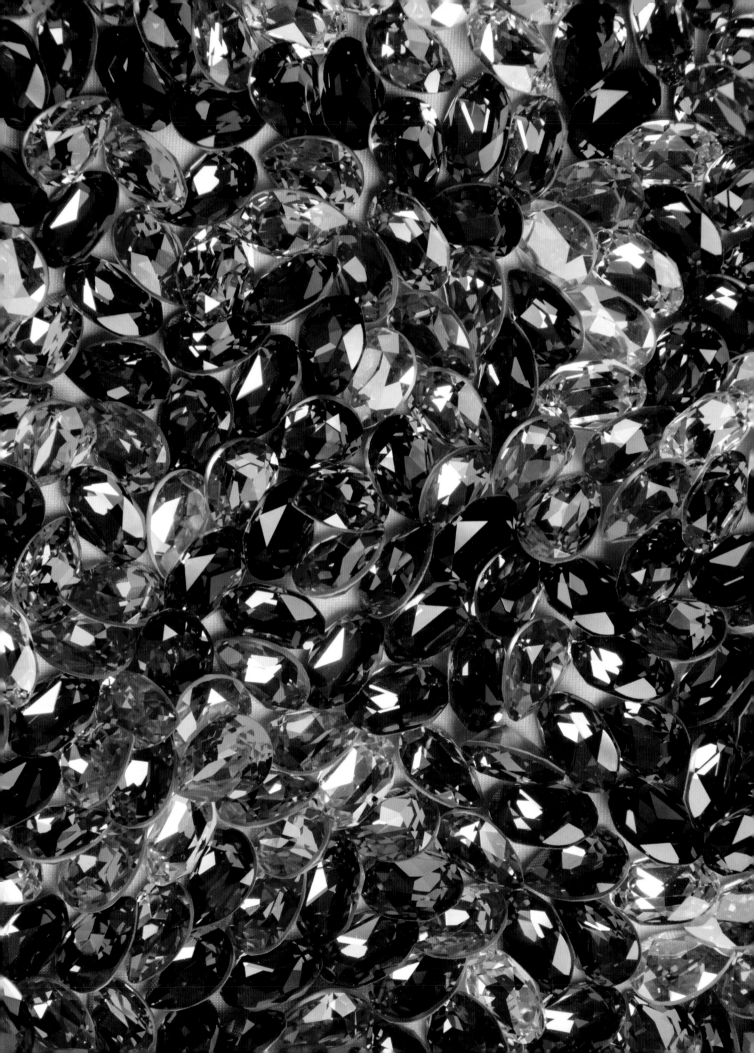

15.
Bling Portfolio

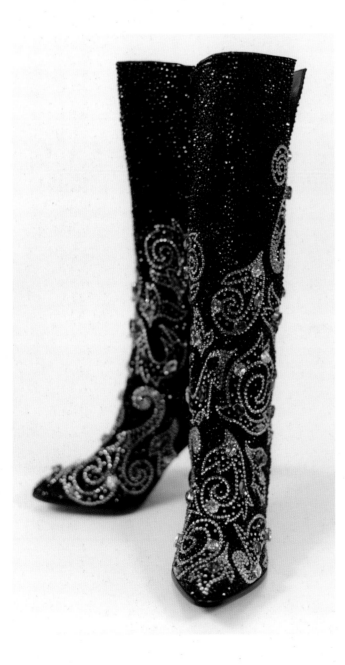

I love what I do! I consider myself one of the luckiest people on the planet to be able to wake up every morning and work at making people happy. I design one-of-a-kind wedding dresses that brides have always dreamed about, and special occasion outfits that grab attention for clients who want to make glamorous entrances. When I make my clients happy, I am happy. The best compliment I ever received was from a client who referred to me as her fairy bling mother.

In this chapter I compiled a portfolio of a few custom pieces ranging from lightly embellished to extravagantly packed with crystals. Perhaps these fanciful creations will inspire you to pick up a bling tool and begin embellishing . . . Enjoy!

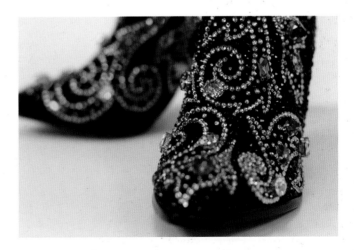

These boots are made for talking! People rave over these knee-high stunners adorned with a total of approximately 60,000 crystals and multicolored fancy stones in gold settings. The swirl design consists of packed Jet and Light Colorado Swarovski® crystals. *Courtesy of Mark Johnson*

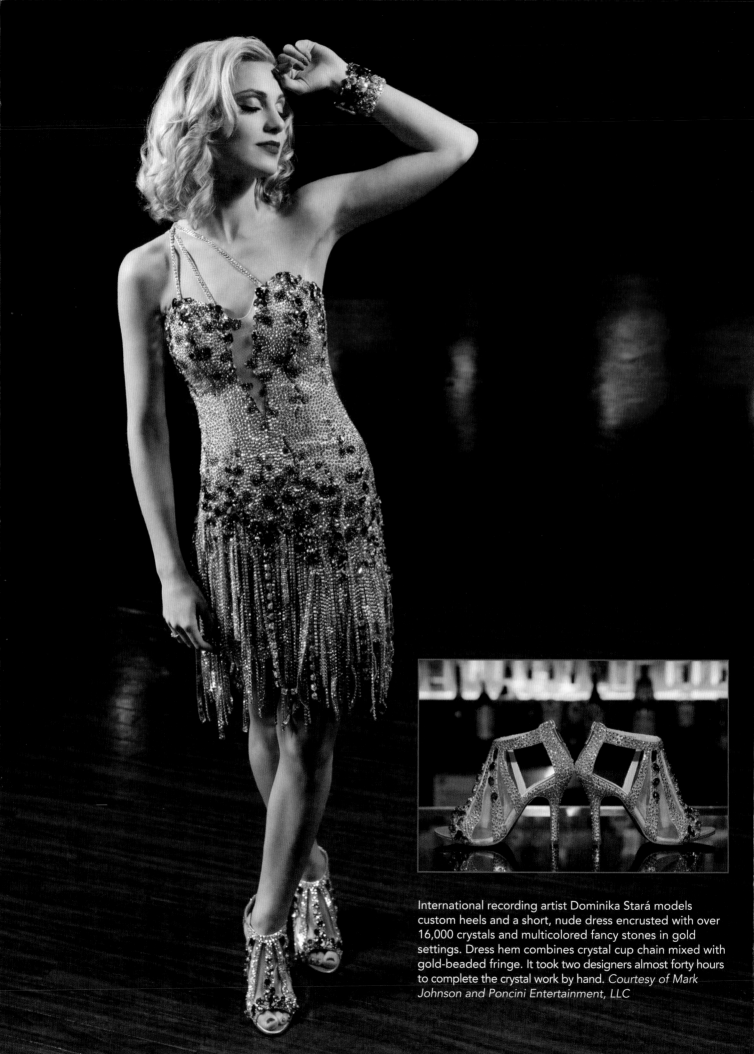

International recording artist Dominika Stará models custom heels and a short, nude dress encrusted with over 16,000 crystals and multicolored fancy stones in gold settings. Dress hem combines crystal cup chain mixed with gold-beaded fringe. It took two designers almost forty hours to complete the crystal work by hand. *Courtesy of Mark Johnson and Poncini Entertainment, LLC*

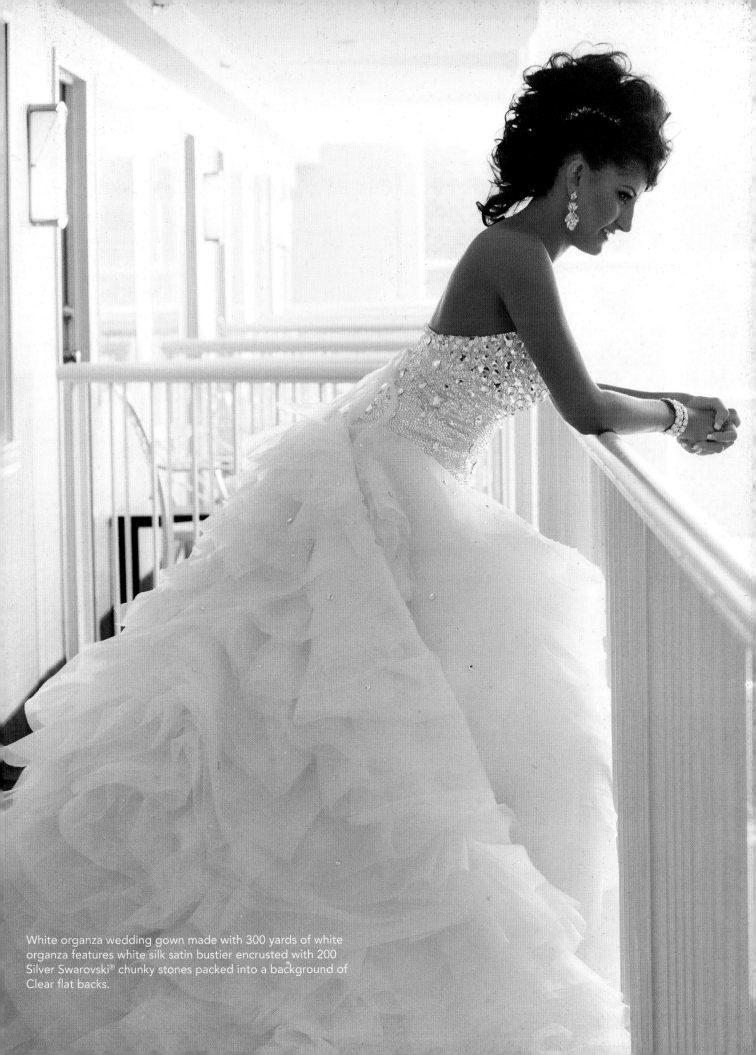

White organza wedding gown made with 300 yards of white organza features white silk satin bustier encrusted with 200 Silver Swarovski® chunky stones packed into a background of Clear flat backs.

Party all night long! Stunning aqua-blue silk organza and tulle party dress embellished with silver guipure lace embellished with Aurora Borealis flat-back stones. Aurora Borealis belt trimmed with matching ornamentation. *Courtesy of Mark Johnson*

Opposite top Personalized iPad covered with thousands of Swarovski® crystals. Three different sizes of flat-back stones in Jet and Clear were used. *Courtesy of Mark Johnson*

Opposite bottom Wild zebra backpack with hot pink accents loaded with almost 70,000 Swarovski® crystals in Jet and Crystal. *Courtesy of Mark Johnson*

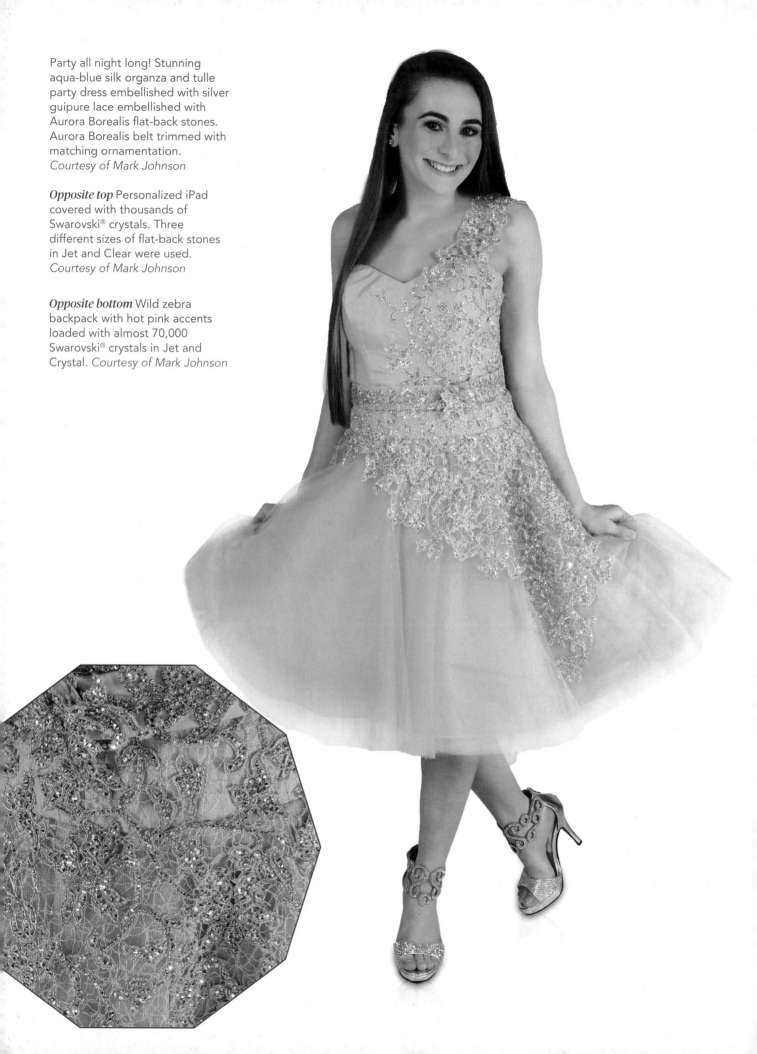

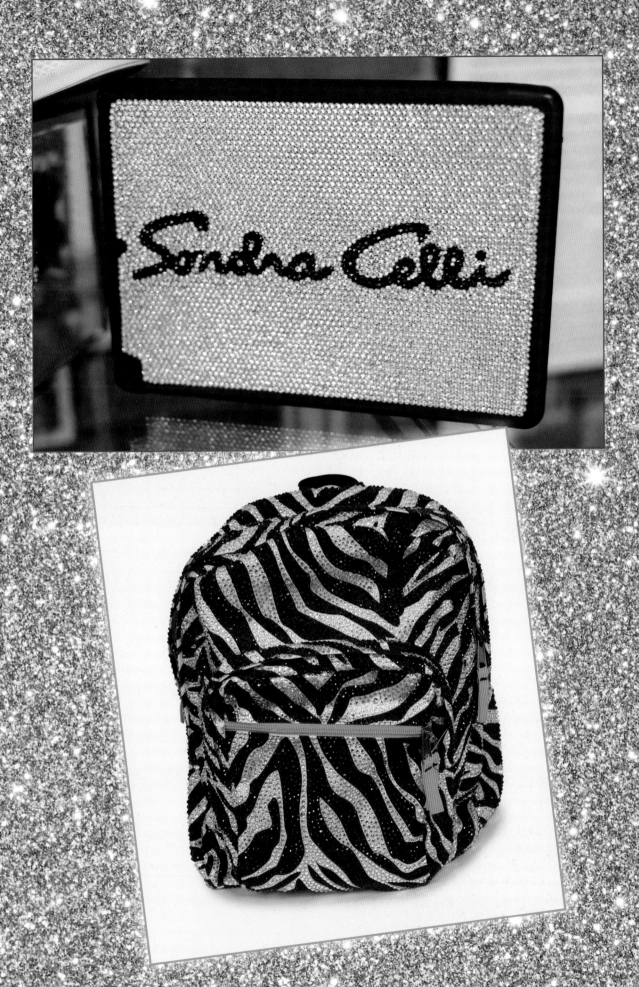

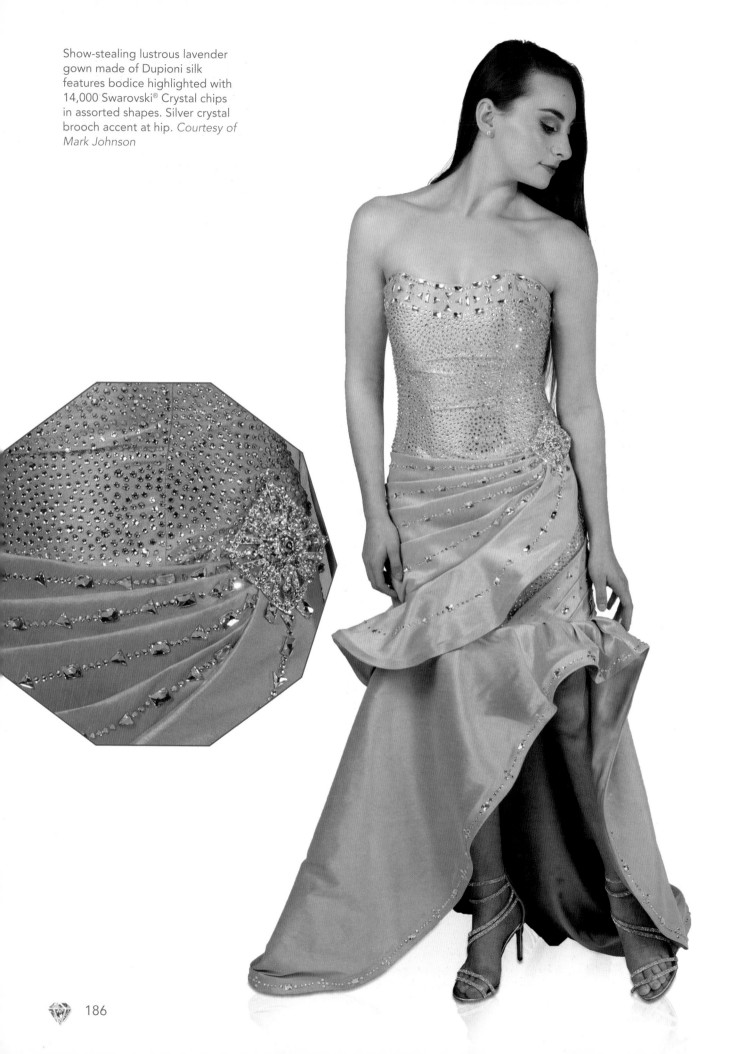

Show-stealing lustrous lavender gown made of Dupioni silk features bodice highlighted with 14,000 Swarovski® Crystal chips in assorted shapes. Silver crystal brooch accent at hip. *Courtesy of Mark Johnson*

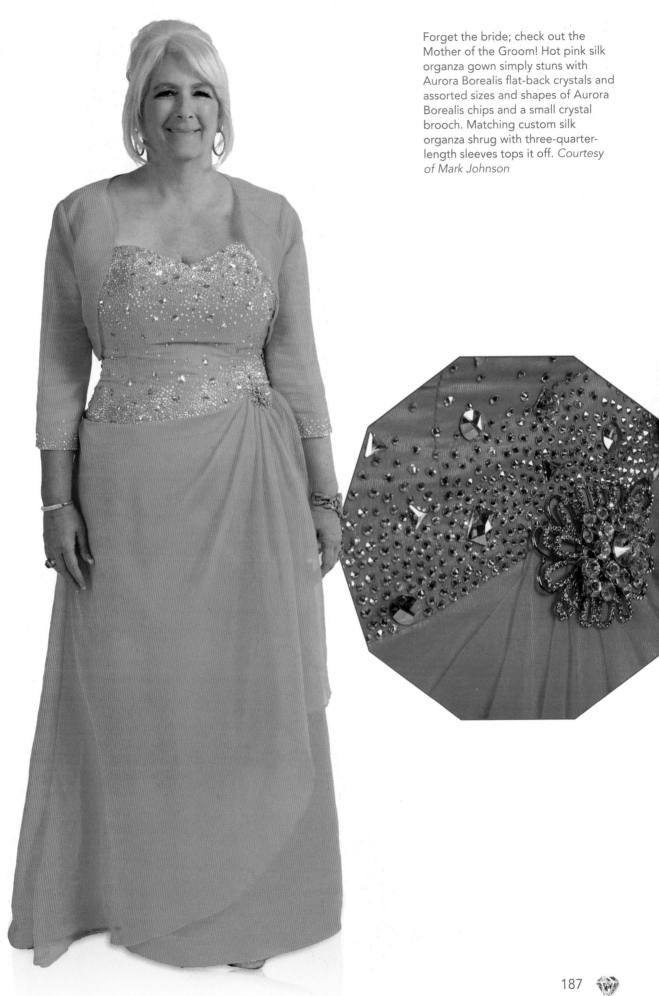

Forget the bride; check out the Mother of the Groom! Hot pink silk organza gown simply stuns with Aurora Borealis flat-back crystals and assorted sizes and shapes of Aurora Borealis chips and a small crystal brooch. Matching custom silk organza shrug with three-quarter-length sleeves tops it off. *Courtesy of Mark Johnson*

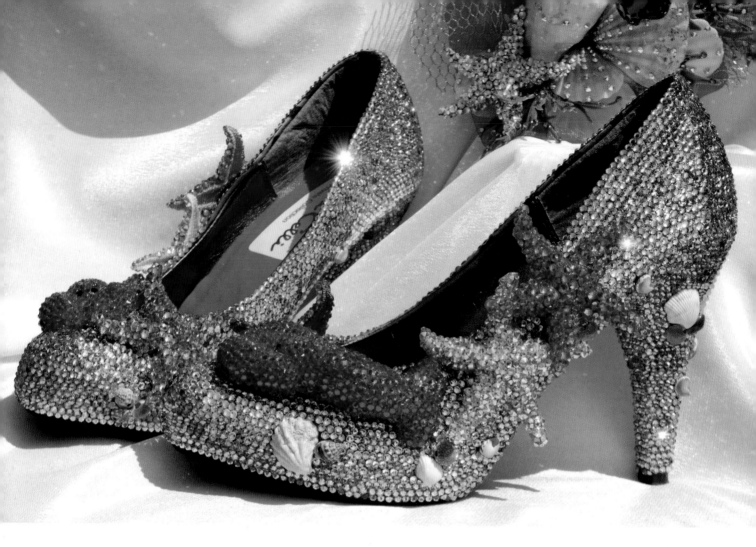

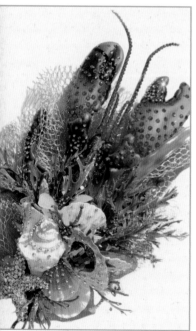

Above and left Reflections of Maine abound in custom heels and matching headpiece worn by Miss Maine at the Show Us Your Shoes Parade, 2013. Aquatic-themed embellishments include crystal-packed lobsters, starfish, authentic seashells, and gold Russian veiling. The 3-D shoe-seascape features a crystal lighthouse up the back of the heels. *Courtesy of Tisi Farrar*

Below Everybody dance now! Bridal bling in the form of sneakers personalized with wedding date and "I Do!" Approximately 14,000 Swarovski crystals in Clear and Light Siam pack the pair. *Courtesy of Lighthouse Photography, www.lighthousephotography.com*

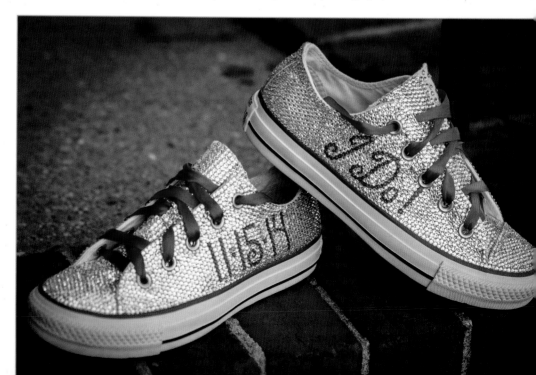

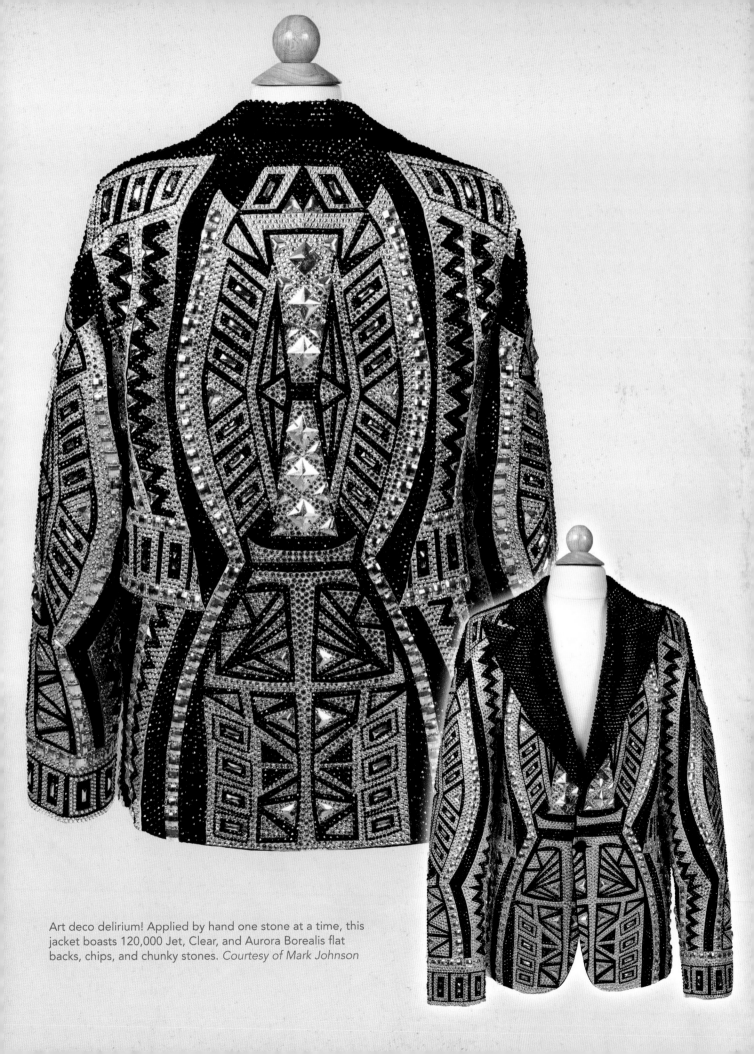

Art deco delirium! Applied by hand one stone at a time, this jacket boasts 120,000 Jet, Clear, and Aurora Borealis flat backs, chips, and chunky stones. *Courtesy of Mark Johnson*

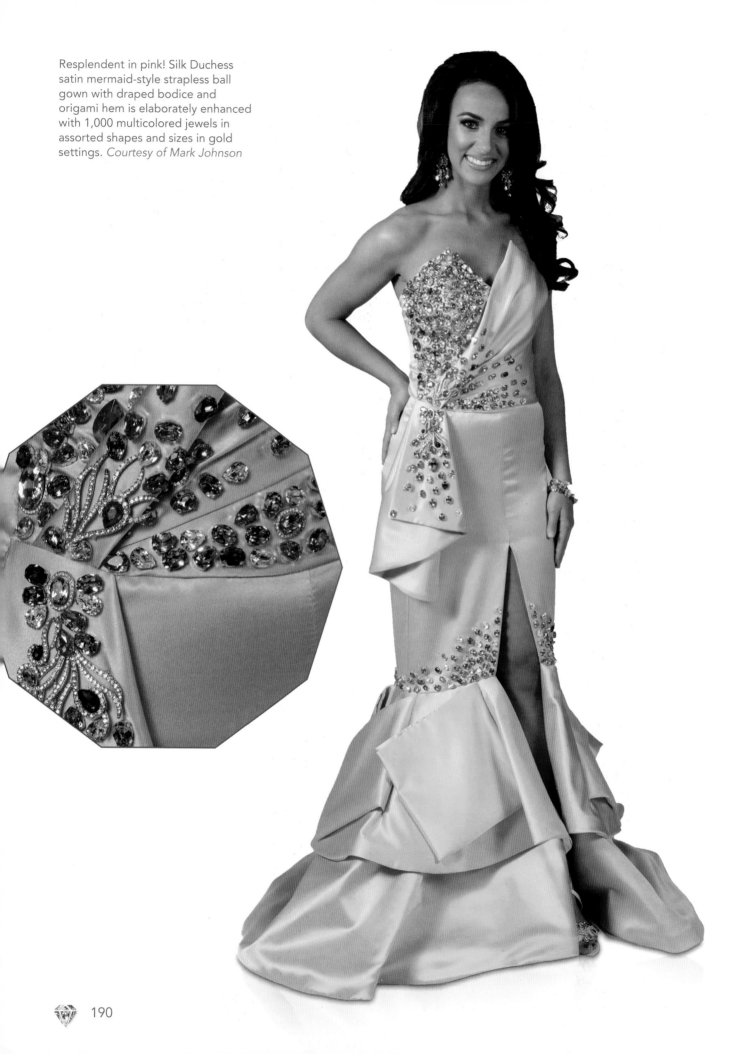

Resplendent in pink! Silk Duchess satin mermaid-style strapless ball gown with draped bodice and origami hem is elaborately enhanced with 1,000 multicolored jewels in assorted shapes and sizes in gold settings. *Courtesy of Mark Johnson*

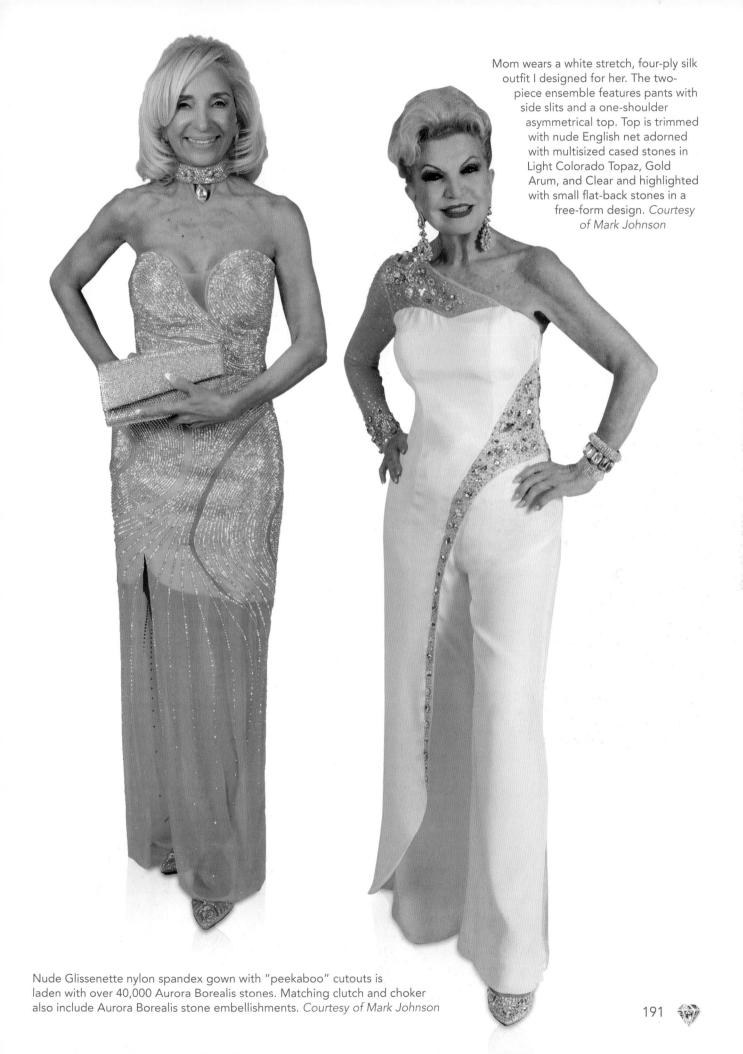

Mom wears a white stretch, four-ply silk outfit I designed for her. The two-piece ensemble features pants with side slits and a one-shoulder asymmetrical top. Top is trimmed with nude English net adorned with multisized cased stones in Light Colorado Topaz, Gold Arum, and Clear and highlighted with small flat-back stones in a free-form design. *Courtesy of Mark Johnson*

Nude Glissenette nylon spandex gown with "peekaboo" cutouts is laden with over 40,000 Aurora Borealis stones. Matching clutch and choker also include Aurora Borealis stone embellishments. *Courtesy of Mark Johnson*

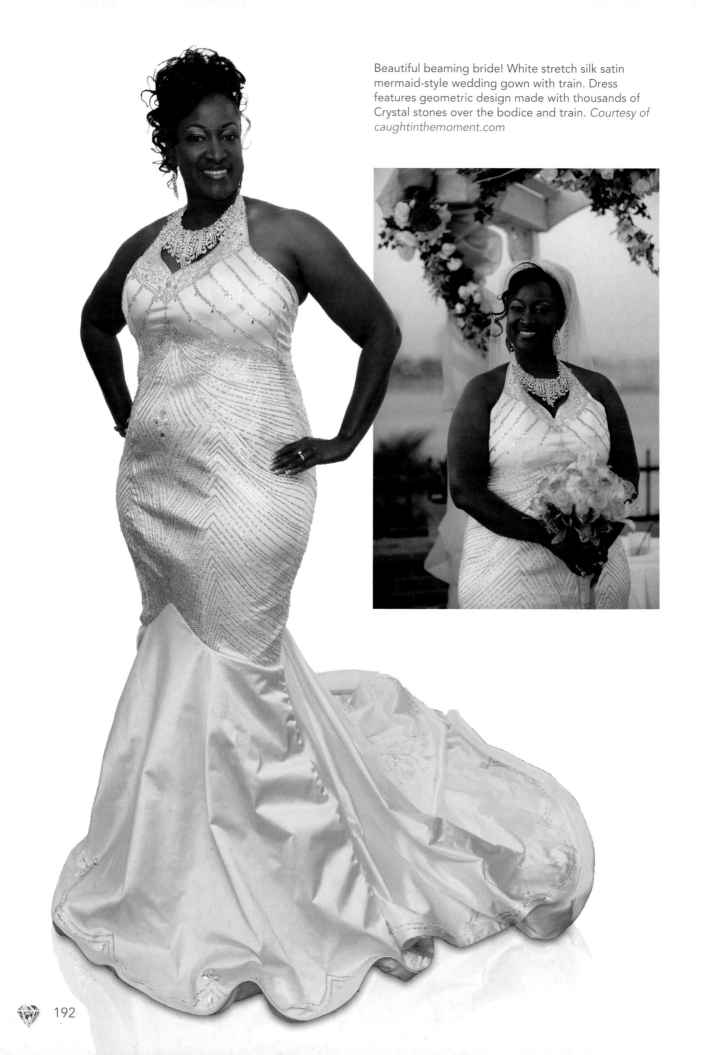

Beautiful beaming bride! White stretch silk satin mermaid-style wedding gown with train. Dress features geometric design made with thousands of Crystal stones over the bodice and train. *Courtesy of caughtinthemoment.com*

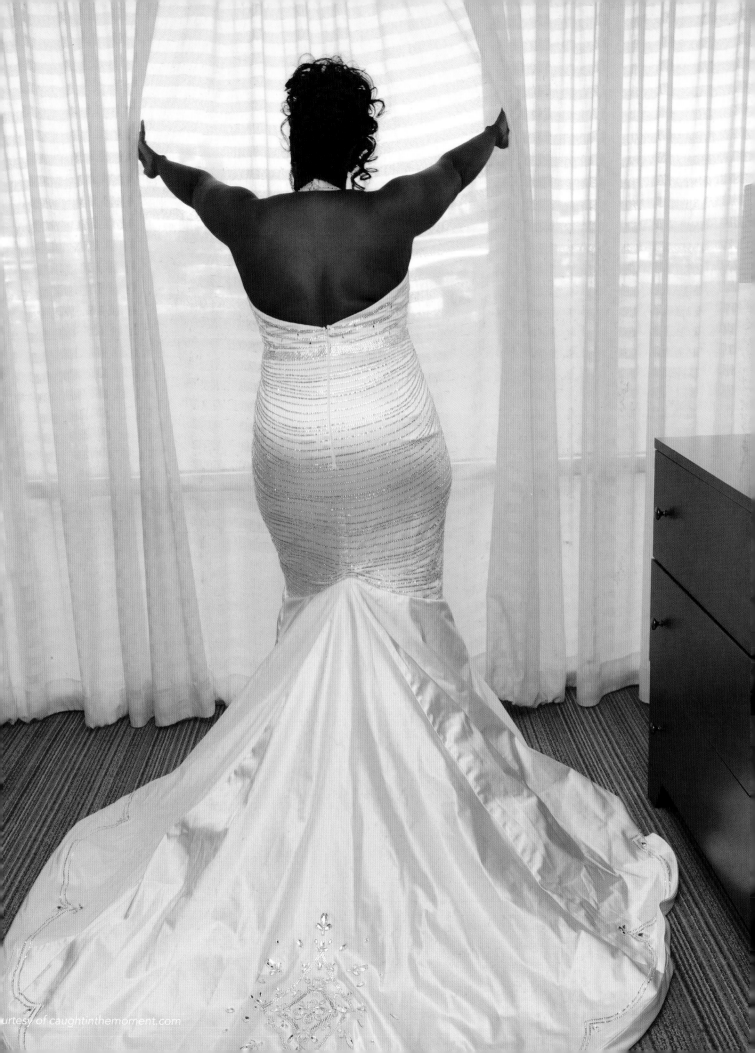

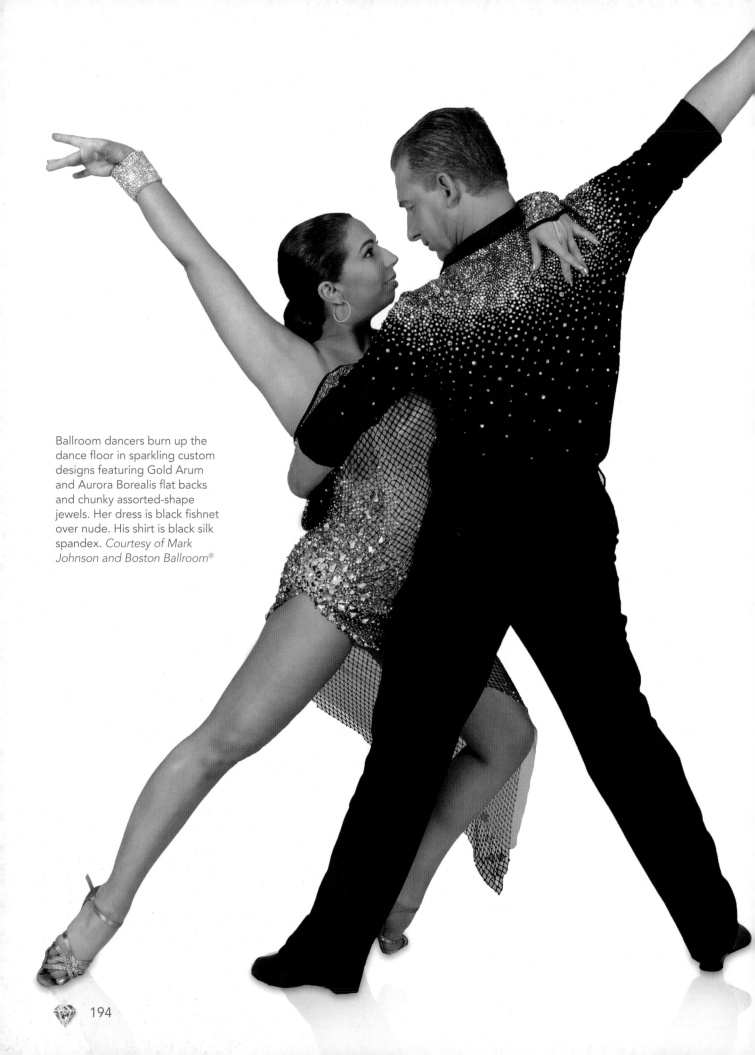

Ballroom dancers burn up the dance floor in sparkling custom designs featuring Gold Arum and Aurora Borealis flat backs and chunky assorted-shape jewels. Her dress is black fishnet over nude. His shirt is black silk spandex. *Courtesy of Mark Johnson and Boston Ballroom®*

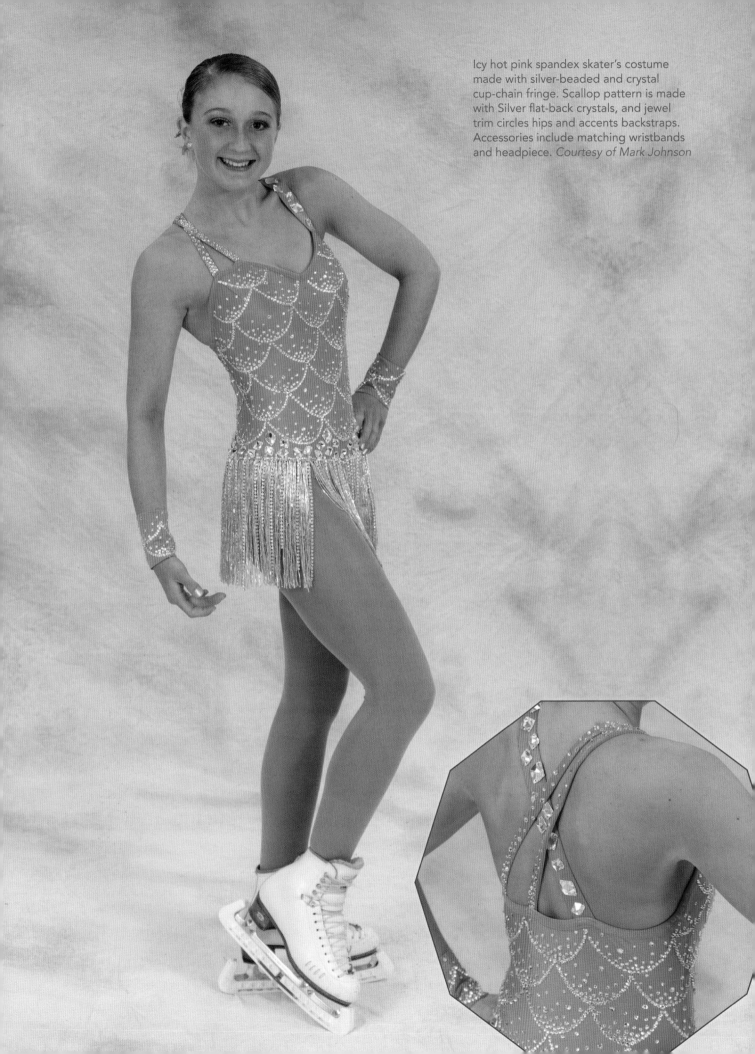

Icy hot pink spandex skater's costume made with silver-beaded and crystal cup-chain fringe. Scallop pattern is made with Silver flat-back crystals, and jewel trim circles hips and accents backstraps. Accessories include matching wristbands and headpiece. *Courtesy of Mark Johnson*

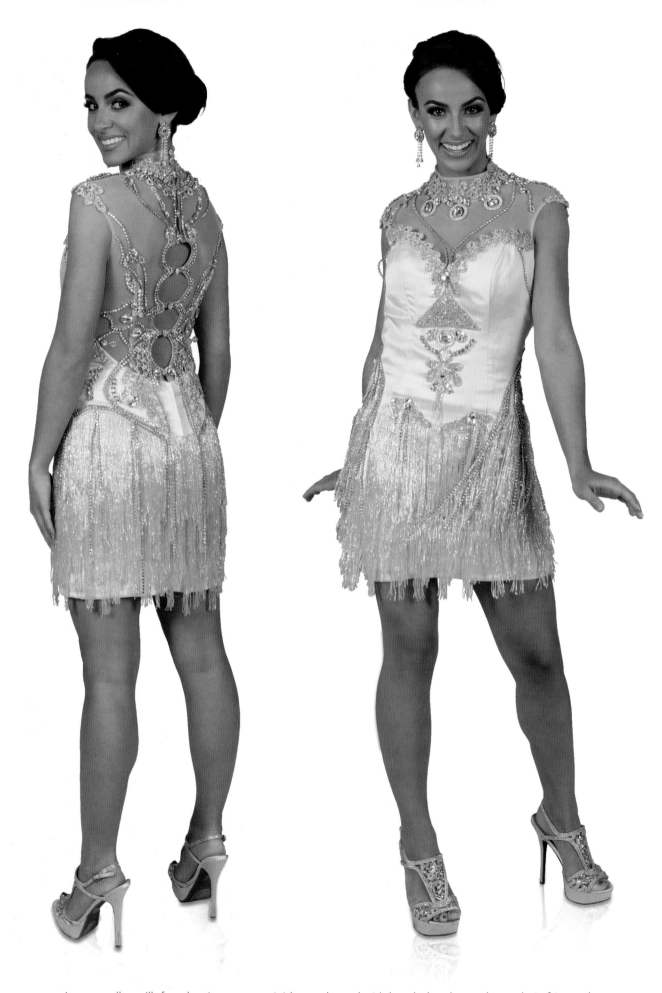

Lemon-yellow silk-faced satin organza minidress adorned with beaded and crystal cup-chain fringe plus assorted broken jewelry pieces: earrings, pendants, necklaces, and bracelets. Sexy sheer back features additional cup-chain fringe trim. *Courtesy of Mark Johnson*

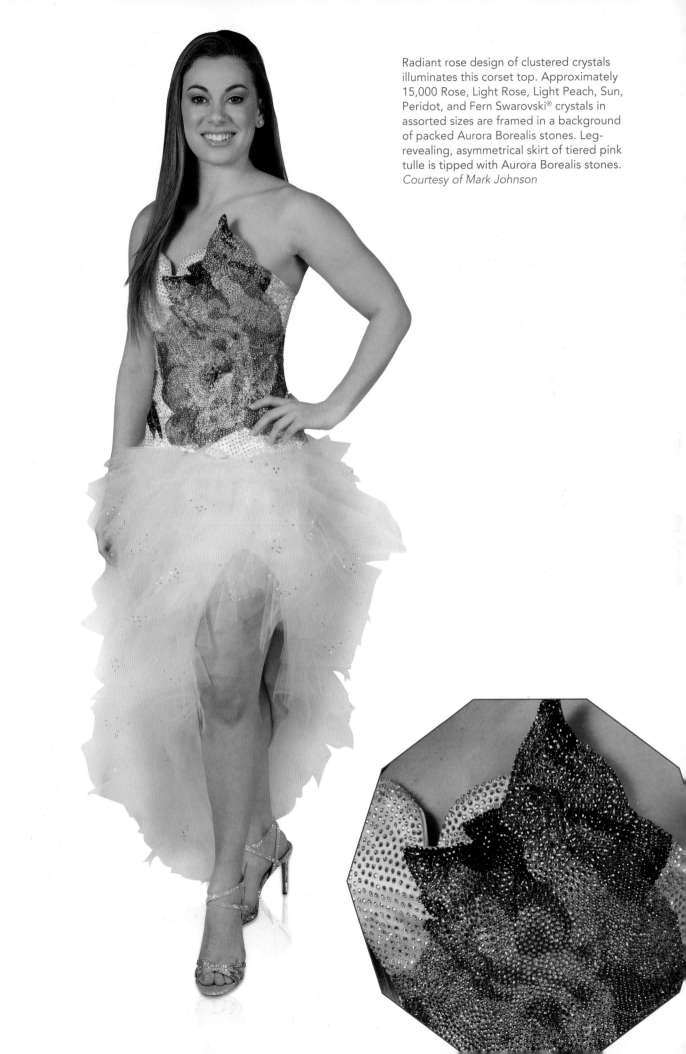

Radiant rose design of clustered crystals illuminates this corset top. Approximately 15,000 Rose, Light Rose, Light Peach, Sun, Peridot, and Fern Swarovski® crystals in assorted sizes are framed in a background of packed Aurora Borealis stones. Leg-revealing, asymmetrical skirt of tiered pink tulle is tipped with Aurora Borealis stones.
Courtesy of Mark Johnson

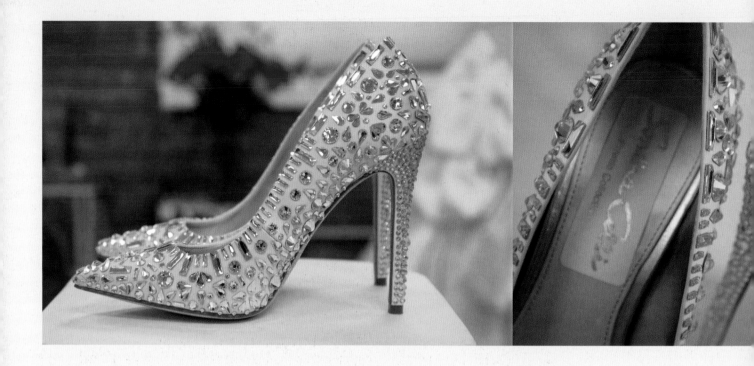

Glass slipper or shimmering pavé heels? Fancy footwear of unmatched brilliance is created with an assortment of Swarovski® Crystal chip stones and flat backs in various shapes and sizes. *Courtesy of Mark Johnson*

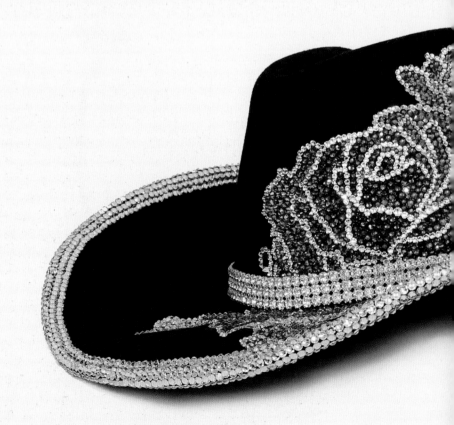

Western wow! Swarovski®-packed trio features boots, belt, and hat. Boots emblazoned with 63,000 Jet Hematite crystals in colors of Volcano, Clear, Fern, Peridot, and Crystal Light. *Courtesy of Mark Johnson*

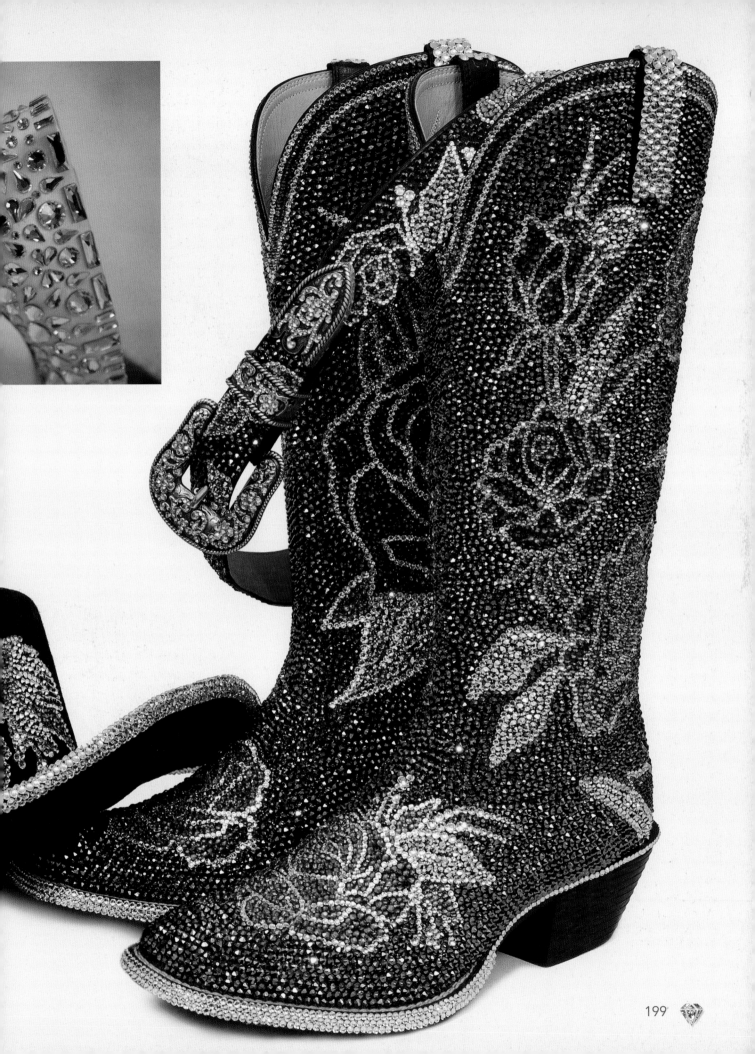

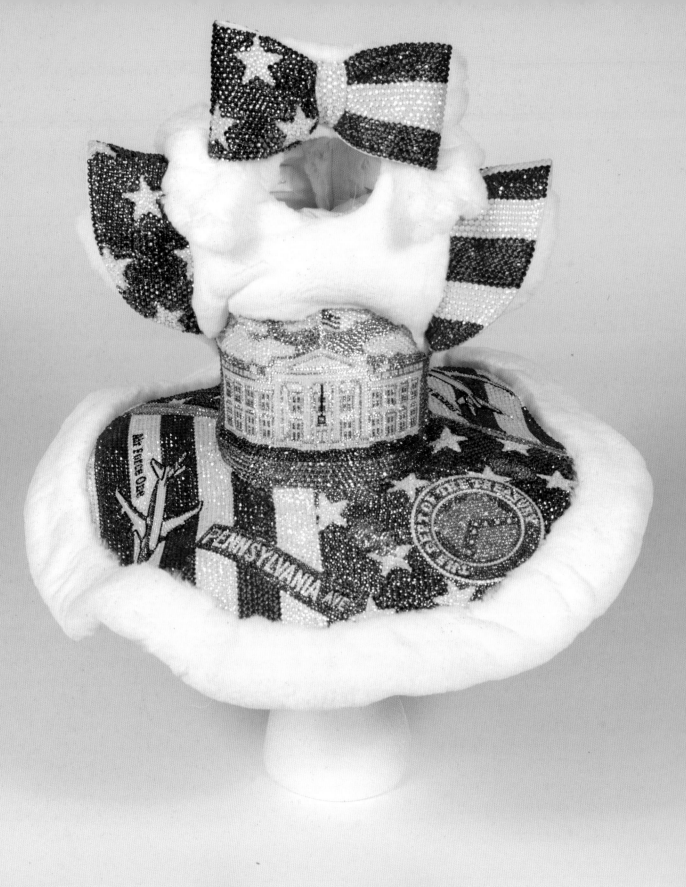
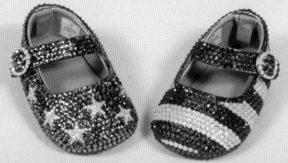

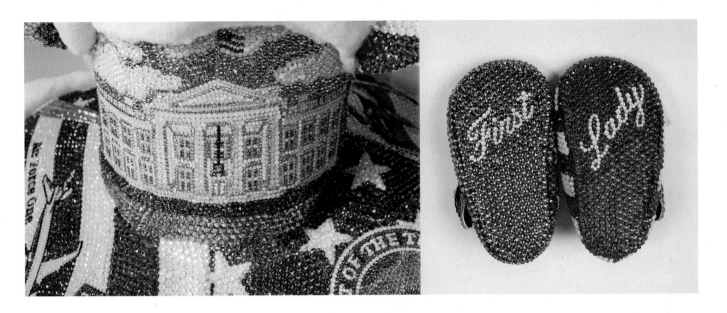

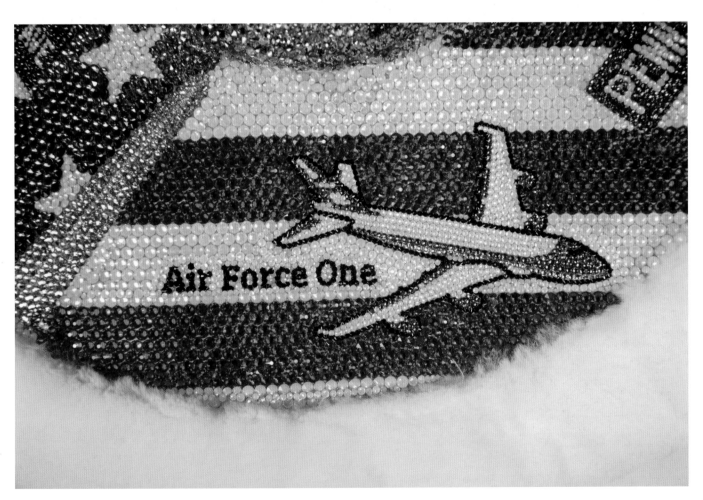

Opposite and above First Baby of Bling! This opulent one-of-a-kind dress features iconic presidential images and is embellished with Light Siam, White Opal, Sapphire, Fern, Peridot, Light Colorado, Light Sapphire, and Jet stones. Over 100,000 stones were used to complete the ensemble, which features matching headband and "First Lady" shoes. *Courtesy of Mark Johnson*

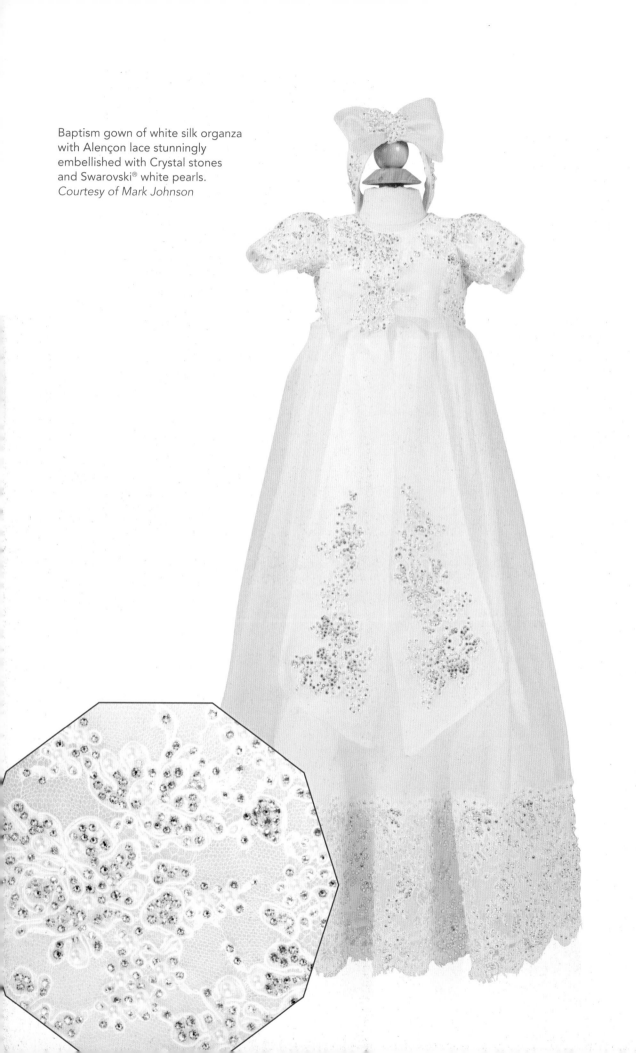

Baptism gown of white silk organza with Alençon lace stunningly embellished with Crystal stones and Swarovski® white pearls.
Courtesy of Mark Johnson

Queenly quinceañera gown made with
300 yards of pink silk organza features
cascading ruffled skirt and lace-up-the-
back corset. Swirl pattern on corset
created with Aurora Borealis flat backs
and chip stones. Miniature version of
dress made for celebrant's baby sister.
Courtesy of www.bodasmodernas.com

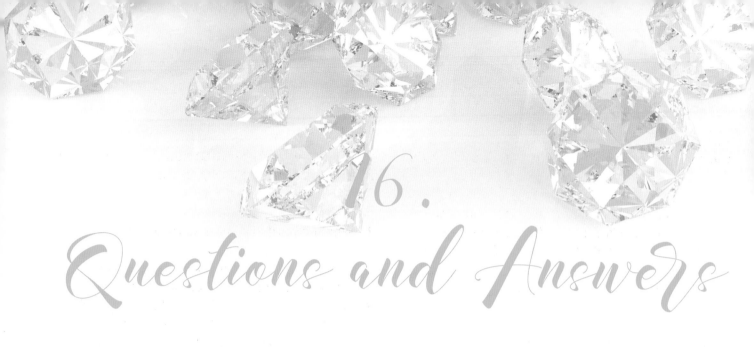

16.
Questions and Answers

This chapter is dedicated to answering many of the most-common questions I get from fans, bling enthusiasts, and clients.

Question: How much time does it take to create a Gypsy wedding gown?

Answer: It depends on the style of dress and the amount of bling. When we tape the show we are usually given just a few days because of the fast-paced production schedule. That's when we have all hands on deck and work around the clock to make the deadline. However, we usually require four to six months to make wedding gowns for clients.

Question: Have you ever had a bride who was unhappy with her gown?

Answer: No, thank goodness. I avoid that by keeping the bride posted as to the progress of the dress from design to assembly and embellishment. I also send photos throughout the process so that there are no unexpected surprises for either of us.

Question: Do you have a favorite design?

Answer: My favorite design is always the one I am currently working on. I get so wrapped up in the creation of it, carefully overseeing each step of the process, down to the exact stone placement. When I finish one project I can hardly wait to get started on the next.

Question: How many people does it take to bling out a Gypsy-style dress?

Answer: It usually takes only one person to add crystals to a dress because the Bling-ettes are crystal design experts. However, when a dress is packed with stones or an intricate design is involved, then it can sometimes take one person three to four weeks to complete just the bling work. One of our biggest designs required twelve of my staff to work on a dress at the same time. We spread the dress out on a work table, and each person had an area to bling out, which helped us finish the work on time.

Question: If you had to choose a different career path tomorrow, what would you choose to do?

Answer: If I were not a designer, I would have been a chef. I love to cook. My favorite thing to make is cheesecake. I can make about twenty-five different flavors of cheesecake without following a recipe. I make them for visitors to my shop (if I know they are coming), for special family gatherings, and for my staff, including the production crew for *My Big Fat American Gypsy Wedding.* In fact, the crew usually calls ahead to order their favorite flavor so that it's on hand for their arrival.

Question: Where do you get your inspiration when designing for clients?

Answer: My design inspiration comes from many different sources: nature, architecture, art, dreams, travel, food, and even a box of crayons. I'm very sensitive to design, color, composition, and texture when I look at things. I also love to challenge myself and try out new concepts.

Question: What is the most frustrating part about being a designer?

Answer: I would have to say it's when I am close to finishing a design and the client starts to second-guess their decisions, wanting to add more elements or to completely change the original design when most of the work has been done. Thank goodness that doesn't happen often, because I keep my clients posted throughout the design process to avoid just such a situation.

Question: Do you ship your designs to other countries?

Answer: I can ship overseas, but international shipping charges can be expensive. For example, a Gypsy-style dress is so big and heavy we usually need to ship it out in two boxes. The cost of shipping is based on the weight and size of the boxes plus destination. At times shipping has run over $300 for each box to an international destination.

Question: What measurements do you require when you have a dress custom designed?

Answer: I need the typical bust, waist, and hip measurements plus the length from the front of your throat (at the indentation) to where you want the hem to fall. In addition, I need the length from bust to waist and bust to hip. Finally, I need a bra size. I also like to request a head-to-toe photo along with the measurements. Combining all that information allows me to create a perfectly fitted design for a client, even when my clients live out of state or out of the country. As long as the measurements I receive are accurate, I can design for anyone without meeting them in person.

Question: Do you design shoes and accessories?

Answer: I don't actually manufacture shoes, but I can custom embellish a pair to match any outfit. We usually ask clients to ship a pair of shoes that they purchase so that they are happy with the heel height, fit, and comfort. We can then custom bling them or add other embellishments such as flowers to match any dress design. Other accessories we can customize include clutches, hair pieces, gloves, jewelry, bouquets, masquerade masks, and more.

Question: Why does a custom design cost so much?

Answer: Clothing that is mass-manufactured in factories by machines can be churned out by the hundreds of thousands every day. When I create a custom piece I must first draft an original pattern based on a person's specific measurements. We also use the best-quality fabrics and finest of crystals, which cost more. All the fabric is cut by hand, sewn together by hand or machine, and embellished by hand–one stone at a time. My staff is made up of veteran designers and expert craftsmen who all receive a living wage. When you purchase one of my custom designs, you are receiving a top-quality product proudly made in America by a stellar artistic team, many of whom have been working in the world of fashion for decades.

Question: Are there ways to save on a custom design?

Answer: Sure! You can select a simple rather than an intricate design, since the more parts a design has, the more time it takes to make, and the higher the cost. Also, select more-affordable fabrics such as tulle and have your design trimmed rather than packed with stones. If you place your order well in advance, you can also save on shipping charges. Finally, if you purchase a store-bought dress on sale, we can always add crystals or other embellishments to give it more life.

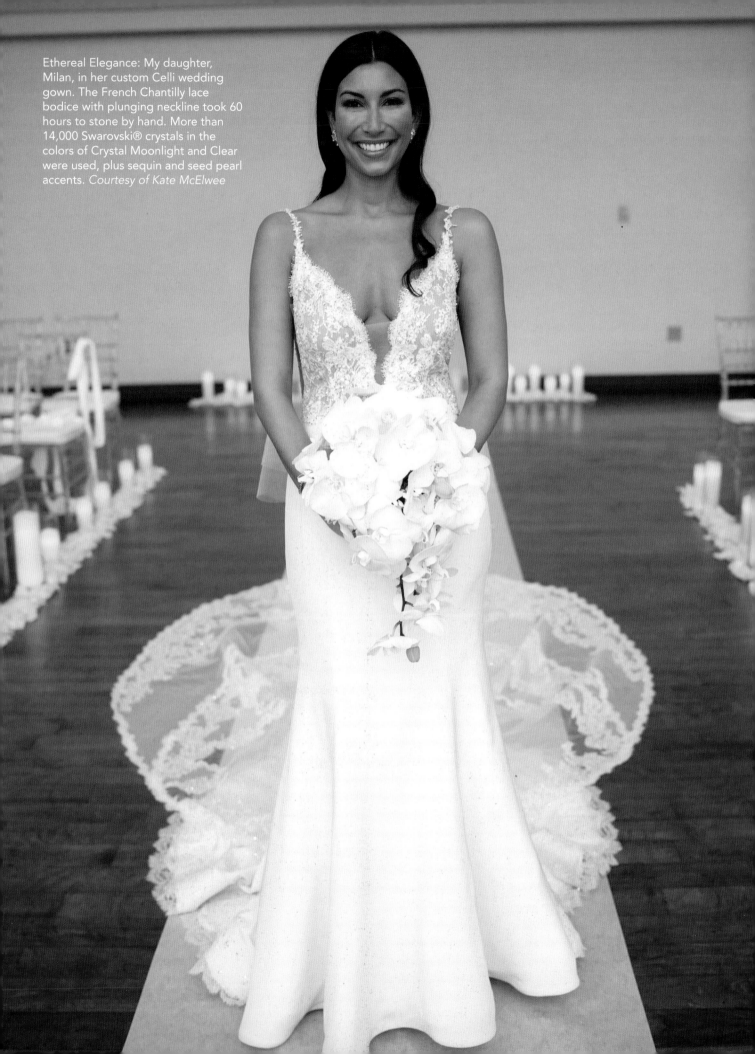

Ethereal Elegance: My daughter, Milan, in her custom Celli wedding gown. The French Chantilly lace bodice with plunging neckline took 60 hours to stone by hand. More than 14,000 Swarovski® crystals in the colors of Crystal Moonlight and Clear were used, plus sequin and seed pearl accents. *Courtesy of Kate McElwee*

Question: What's the craziest dress you have ever designed?

Answer: I have made quite a few crazy designs over the years, but one that sticks out is the dress made up entirely of wigs. A client wanted a short, sexy dress made from wigs. I ordered in a number of long-haired black and white wigs and just clipped off the scalp area to open them up and then sewed them together as if they were yards of fringe. Not only was the client thrilled with the design, she saved on dry-cleaning bills since she could simply wear it into the shower and give it a good shampoo! (Just kidding.)

Question: Has there ever been a design request that you've had to turn down?

Answer: No. Somehow I always figure it out no matter how bizarre the request.

Question: How do you clean a dress embellished with crystals?

Answer: The only way to clean a dress made with authentic crystals is to have it professionally spot cleaned. It should not be washed or dry-cleaned, because those methods can affect the quality of the adhesive and cause stones to fall off.

Question: Do you have a favorite client?

Answer: Yes—my daughter, Milan. I have been creating custom designs for her since she was born. She is also my toughest client. She was recently married, and I'm glad to say that she was absolutely thrilled with the wedding dress and reception ensemble that I designed for her.

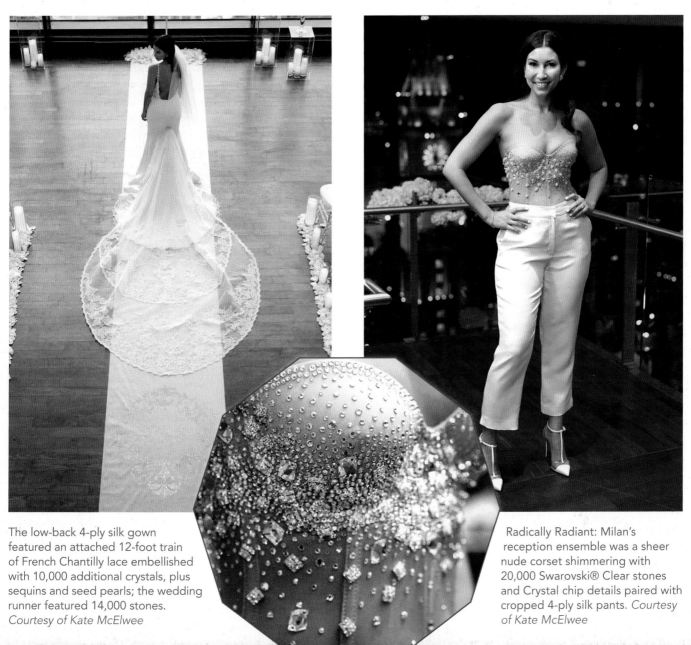

The low-back 4-ply silk gown featured an attached 12-foot train of French Chantilly lace embellished with 10,000 additional crystals, plus sequins and seed pearls; the wedding runner featured 14,000 stones. *Courtesy of Kate McElwee*

Radically Radiant: Milan's reception ensemble was a sheer nude corset shimmering with 20,000 Swarovski® Clear stones and Crystal chip details paired with cropped 4-ply silk pants. *Courtesy of Kate McElwee*

About the Authors

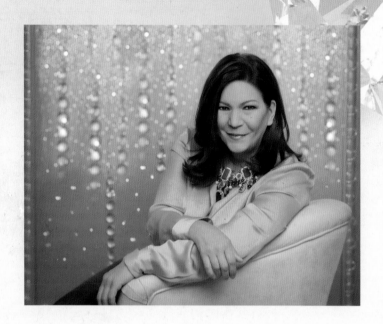

World-renowned crystal couture designer and popular television personality **Sondra Celli** is a graduate of New York's Fashion Institute of Technology (FIT). She apprenticed in Italy, France, England, Switzerland, Sweden, and Denmark, then went on to work at several prestigious fashion houses in New York, Italy, and Hong Kong, earning numerous awards along the way. In 1981 she established the Sondra Celli Company, designing uncommon crystal couture for infants, children, and women of all ages, shapes, and sizes.

Sondra's imaginative creations have been seen in *Vogue, Town & Country, Harper's Bazaar, New York Magazine*, the *New York Times, Modern Bride*, the *Boston Globe, The Sun*, and the *Huffington Post*. Her television features include the series *Gypsy Sisters* and the series special *Bling It On*. In addition, Sondra's more whimsical designs and over-the-top wedding dresses have been showcased on the hit series *My Big Fat American Gypsy Wedding*.

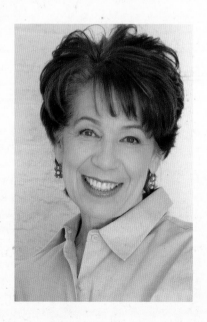

Former television producer **Tisi Farrar** has worked behind the scenes for over 30 years on major network talk shows, live event productions, and awards specials. She currently works as director of marketing and media relations for Sondra Celli Company and is known for sporting a pair of custom bling glasses while she works.

Photo courtesy of Rachael Lynsey Rubin